Tongue Tied

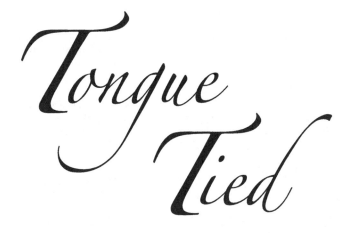

Tongue Tied

UNTANGLING COMMUNICATION IN
SEX, KINK, AND RELATIONSHIPS

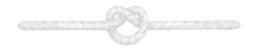

STELLA HARRIS

CLEiS
PRESS

Published in the United States by Cleis Press, an imprint of Start Midnight, LLC, 101 Hudson Street, Thirty-Seventh Floor, Suite 3705, Jersey City, NJ 07302.

Printed in the United States
Cover design: Allyson Fields
Cover photograph: iStock
Text design: Frank Wiedemann

First Edition.
10 9 8 7 6 5 4 3 2 1

Trade paper ISBN: 978-1-62778-266-1
E-book ISBN: 978-1-62778-267-8

Library of Congress Cataloging-in-Publication Data is available on file.

TABLE OF CONTENTS

ACKNOWLEDGMENTS

IN A LOT OF WAYS, I'VE BEEN REALLY LUCKY. I'VE had amazing people in my life—many who showed up at just the right time—who have helped me learn about sex, love, relationships, kink, communication, and more. As early as middle school, I was fascinated by sex, poring over the anatomy sections of the encyclopedia and dog-earing the pages where sex scenes happened in the paperbacks I was reading.

By late high school, when I started exploring with other people, I was incredibly lucky to find partners who were open-minded and contributed to my education. My first serious boyfriend gave me the books *Screw the Roses, Send Me the Thorns* and *Bi Any Other Name,* books that influenced my early education in kink and sexuality and showed me that I wasn't alone.

At seventeen I started attending local munches in West Hollywood, which were held in coffee shops and open to all ages, as well as local poly and bisexual meet-up groups. I was lucky that I lived in LA, and in such a big city there were meet-ups for everything. The people I met at those groups had a big influence on me, and some of them are still friends today.

The thing that really blew me away about these communities was how well everyone communicated. It quickly became clear that to do these activities well, and safely, good communication was a must.

Aside from liking the kinky sex and the open relationships, I felt at ease with these people because I knew I could trust them to say what they meant. That was the norm for me for so long that when I was finally out of school and in an office environment, I was utterly baffled by the complete lack of communication skills people demonstrated. People were passive-aggressive and manipulative. People didn't speak to each other directly but instead complained about coworkers behind their backs. It was unbearable.

After a decade behind a desk, I became a full-time sex educator and I was back among my people—back in spaces where I knew people would speak up about their needs, not just in sexual situations, but in professional and interpersonal situations, too.

In the field of sex, kink, and relationships, I've attended numerous conferences, classes, trainings, and seminars, and I've read more books than I can possibly count. I've had amazing friends and colleagues I've learned from and workshopped ideas with. I know that I've sponged up ideas from every partner I've ever had, every class I've taken, and every book I've read.

As I've worked on this book, the generosity of my friends has blown me away. Everyone has been willing to brainstorm, talk, share their stories, and give me encouragement. One friend even let me stick Post-It notes all over her house. And while I couldn't have done it without my whole community, I want to give special thanks to my coworking group, my mastermind group, and every friend, teacher, partner, and therapist I've ever had.

Communication skills can't be learned or practiced in a vacuum, and everyone I've ever known has been essential to getting me where I am today.

INTRODUCTION

IN MY YEARS AS A SEX EDUCATOR AND COACH, the number one question and concern I hear is about communication (even when the people asking don't realize it). From not knowing how to bring up vulnerable topics to not having the language for the things they want to try to fearing that talking at all will "ruin the mood."

I hear these things so much that all of my classes—regardless of topic—include segments on communication, and it's a big part of all my private coaching sessions, too. Interested in bondage? You've got to talk about it. Want to open your relationship? So much talking. Eager to try new kinds of sex? You guessed it—that requires a conversation.

Despite how vital communication is to our sexual health and well-being, most people have no idea how to talk about sex, or even bodies. The combination of a lack of factual information, combined with a shroud of shame, leaves many people paralyzed.

I got a stark lesson in just how uninformed people are about bodies when I was only thirteen years old. My sex-positive mother, who raised me with shame-free and factual information about sex and bodies, passed away, and I moved in with my paternal grandparents. The shame-free information came to a screeching halt.

When I got my period, it was no surprise, because, thankfully, I'd been prepared for that by my mother. So I hopped on my bike, rode to the local drugstore, and got some tampons. Some time later my grandmother saw the tampons and had a fit. While some of her argument had a moralistic tone that I wasn't ready to refute at that age, her argument also had factual inaccuracies that I was ready to point out. She told me that using tampons would break my hymen.

So I used the tools that were available to me in the pre-Internet age, and I pulled out the encyclopedia, turned to the section with the layered transparency pages that showed genital anatomy, and I taught my grandmother about hymens.

That experience left a mark on me, and I've never shaken what it feels like to be shamed for natural things that bodies do, or what it's like to have to confront inaccurate information with your own hard-won knowledge.

These days talking and writing about sex and bodies is my full-time job. I've gotten to a point where it's not just easy, it's second nature. But there's no chance I'll forget how scary it is for most people. I hear that every day from my students and clients. It's a guarantee that every time I teach a class someone will ask, "But won't talking ruin the mood?" My heart breaks for all the people suffering through mediocre sex in silence.

Doesn't bad sex ruin the mood all on its own? Whether it's an oops in a kink scene or a sexual encounter gone sideways, I find it hard to believe mustering the courage for a conversation would be worse.

Sometimes I explain this. Sometimes I demonstrate

dirty talk. Maybe it's because I'm a language nerd, but talking about what we're going to do is one of my biggest turn-ons. When a partner whispers that he's been thinking how good it feels to have his fingers inside me, my pulse quickens. When a partner tells me she can't wait to try out a new toy on me, I tingle just thinking about it. Not only is anticipating what's going to happen part of the fun, but if I don't want that—or I want something else—I have time to say so.

People come to my office and tell me things they've never said out loud before. They tell me their desires, their fetishes, and their fears. They tell me what they'd love to try. And again and again, I tell them they have to talk to their partner. And I give them the tools to do so.

If you're uncomfortable talking about the kind of touch you like, or discussing safer sex needs, what happens if you need to talk about an unexpected pregnancy or a positive STI result? Getting used to talking and having clear and open communication can be a lifesaver when big issues come up, because you already have a framework for having conversations—even difficult or uncomfortable ones.

And while I know people find talking scary, I've seen the breakthroughs my clients have made. I've seen people report back from one coaching session to the next that everything has changed—gotten easier—because they have the words they need now. When I teach at conventions, sex shops, and sex-positive venues, my communication class is a mainstay. That class includes some of the exercises you'll read about in this book.

My favorite thing when I'm working with students or clients is when their eyes go wide with the aha moment that they really can have the sex life of their dreams. It's my hope that with this book, you can as well.

Stella Harris
Portland, Oregon

HOW TO USE THIS BOOK

I SUSPECT YOU'LL USE THIS BOOK, LIKE MOST books of its kind, in two ways. You'll either skim it or read it cover to cover now, when you're first picking it up, and then later you'll use it as a reference when you're addressing a particular issue or new relationship.

I'm a big book nerd, both personally and professionally, and my home and office are filled with books. I'm not sure I have a single book-free surface. And although I have sticky tabs marking my favorite passages, whenever I pick up a beloved reference, I find something new. Maybe the first time I read the book I wasn't dealing with jealousy, but now every word in that section leaps off the page like it was written just for me. That tends to be the way of these things. Some tools don't speak to you until you need them.

The other difference could be whether you read this alone or with a partner. Again, either is fine. Some of the exercises call for self-reflection, and others can be done with a partner, in or out of the bedroom.

With many exercises you could be doing it as a book club for two (or more), where you work through chapters and examples intentionally. But many of the items can also be brought up casually, with no reference to the book. You'll have to get a feel for what style works for you.

In my classes, I always tell students that now they have me as an excuse. If they need an icebreaker with their partner to try something new, or to bring up a touchy subject, they can say, "So I was in this class . . ." Because sometimes knowing how to start the conversation is the hardest part. That's probably one of the reasons you're reading this book. So feel free to use it as your excuse, from mentioning what you're reading to leaving it on the coffee table. This book is a tool, and I encourage you to use it in any or all of the ways that make sense for you and your situation.

UNDERLYING PHILOSOPHIES

This book is written based on some core philosophies. It assumes that we're all responsible for ourselves and the way we behave in relationships, and also for our own well-being and needs. Ultimately we're all responsible for getting our own needs met, from having sex to having orgasms to getting to try that new restaurant that just opened. Would we like our partner(s) to be involved in some or all of those things? Sure. But it's still our responsibility to ask rather than expect them to read our mind.

And if your partner doesn't want to go to that restaurant? That's when you decide if you want to go alone, or with another partner, or with a friend. Or maybe to decide that it wasn't a need but a want, and one you can do without.

The same is true for sex. You can't get what you want if you don't ask for it. So this book will give you ideas of things to ask for, as well as ways to do the asking. But it's always possible the other person will be unable or unwilling to do what you've asked, so then it's up to you to figure out how to take care of yourself in that situation. And we'll talk about that, too—about what to do when you hear "no."

SOME NOTES ON LANGUAGE

You'll read the word *partner* in this book a lot. It's already appeared in this chapter several times. When I use the word *partner*, I mean whoever is in front of you in that moment. It can mean a hookup you'll spend an hour with, and it could mean someone you've committed to spending your life with. It's referring to whomever you're having sex, kink, and conversations with.

The word *negotiation* will also come up in every chapter, if not every page. For some people the term brings up frightful memories of asking for a raise or buying a house. For others, they think of a lose-lose compromise. When I say *negotiation*, I mean a very particular kind of communication used to reach agreements around sex and kink. In sex and kink negotiation, everyone's needs, desires, and limits are taken into account, and the only activities that will be engaged in are the ones everyone feels good about.

Kink refers to a whole range of activities, from spanking to bondage to more advanced fetishes. The term is very versatile and tends to stand in for any activity (usually sexual) that's considered unconventional or outside the mainstream.

I also use the word *play* liberally. It's commonly used in both kink and sex-positive communities to describe the activities two—or more—people are going to engage in. Play could be a threesome, or it could be a spanking. It's a way of defining the set period of time when these activities are being engaged in.

This book also strives to be as gender neutral and sexuality neutral as possible. Unlike some popular books on relationships, I don't believe the genders are all that different. Yes, the way people are socialized is hugely influenced by our presentations. But I don't think treating your partner like an alien, or like an animal to be tamed, is a healthy or productive stance to take.

> *"A study at Rosalind Franklin University of Medicine and Science, led by Lise Eliot, has found that the hippocampus is the same size in both men and women. The team's discovery came from a meta-analysis of more than 6,000 structural MRI scans, which showed that there was 'no significant difference in hippocampal size between men and women.' The discovery also counters many popular explanations of the differences between men and women. 'Sex differences in the brain are irresistible to those looking to explain stereotypic differences between men and women,' said Eliot. 'And they often make a big splash. But as we explore multiple data sets and are able to coalesce very large samples of males and females, we find these differences often disappear or are trivial.' "*
>
> —FROM A *WIRED* ARTICLE
> BY EMILY REYNOLDS[1]

The problems of socialization in a sex-negative society are why this book also talks about figuring out, and owning, your own shit. Have you been socialized as a caretaker?

---

1   Emily Reynolds, "There Probably Is No Such Thing as 'Male' and 'Female' Brain," *Wired UK*, October 30, 2015. http://www.wired.co.uk/article/male-female-brain-difference-not-significant

(I certainly have.) That's something you need to learn about yourself so you can figure out how to balance those impulses with your own self-care. Not to mention avoid stifling another person by providing care they haven't asked for and don't want.

Have you been socialized to believe your needs come first, or that doing the dishes is never your responsibility? That's something to look at, too.

You can negotiate any kind of relationship you want to have. Maybe you fetishize 1950s households, and playing those roles is part of your dynamic. That's fine with me. As long as everything that means to you has been explicitly stated and agreed upon by everyone involved. Because where we get in trouble is when we make assumptions. And many of those assumptions are drilled into us from day one, often based on our perceived genders.

So do the homework of turning those assumptions on their heads, or at least interrogating them so you can keep what's useful to you and discard the rest. Perhaps the only guarantee I can make is that figuring out and owning all of your biases and assumptions will improve your communication and your relationships.

Some writing and advice on relationships would have you waiting for "your other half." As much as I love the Aristophanes myth, I don't buy the story. And I think it's harmful. We're all whole and fully realized people on our own. And maintaining our own identities, and our own independence, is essential for showing up in a healthy way to our relationships.

Whether well meaning or not, sometimes people use tools meant to help with communication or relationships as a way to manipulate others. The way it usually goes is that someone points to the tools or philosophies in the book to tell someone else they're "doing it wrong" or to bring all communication to a halt until it's spoken in the form the book suggests —like the buzzer going off in *Jeopardy!* if you don't answer in the form of a question.

Using the tools in this way utterly misses the point. It's turning them into weapons, and that isn't fair to their creators, or to your partner(s). So use the tools in this book (and others) to improve your communication skills, not to control the behavior of others.

I hope you'll find some of the tools and exercises in this book helpful. But keep in mind that you can choose what's useful to you and leave the rest.

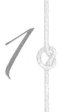 **What Are We Aiming For?**

HEALTHY RELATIONSHIPS AND GOOD COMMUNICATION

> *"The best measure of the health of any relationship is the quality of the communication in it. Every single thing that we can't or won't talk about, openly and without fear or shame, is a crack in the relationship's foundation."*
>
> —FRANKLIN VEAUX AND EVE RICKERT,
> *MORE THAN TWO*

WE ALL WANT TO FEEL HEARD AND UNDERSTOOD. With partners, with friends, with coworkers, communication is essential to human interaction. But just because we've all been practicing it since we uttered our first words doesn't mean we've learned how to communicate effectively.

Especially when it comes to a romantic or sexual relationship, good communication is essential. Most people would agree with that, but when you dig down into details and applications, it gets a little trickier.

So what does good communication in a relationship mean? It means when you speak you feel heard. It means each person in the relationship has empathy for their partner, and everyone has both their own and the other person—or people's—well-being in mind. It means feeling safe bringing up your feelings, fears, wants, and desires. Knowing that when you speak up you won't be criticized, judged, or shamed. That you have a safe space to share what's going on with you, and that you'll truly be listened to and understood.

Talking, confiding, sharing—it all builds trust.

Think about your earliest friendships, when you were a kid. Sharing secrets was one of the biggest signs of close friendship. We'd whisper or pass notes, and these confidences were shared with only our closest friends. Hopefully our communication styles have grown a bit since those days, but the essentials are the same: we feel the closest to the people we feel most comfortable sharing with.

And to be fair, maybe some of it hasn't changed that much. Where once we passed notes in the halls, now we might exchange text messages. Instead of whispering to someone under the covers with flashlights lighting your face, we have postsex pillow talk. But one thing remains the same—these are the ways we experience intimacy.

Think about how you felt the first time someone leaned over and whispered, "Can I tell you a secret?" Do you remember the rush of excitement? The feeling you got because someone trusted you that much? And not only that, but how eager you were to hear what they were going to tell you?

Our secrets may have changed, but we can recapture those feelings in our adult lives, too. That exchange of vulnerability. Giving another person the chance to reject or accept us, and thrilling when the new information we've shared brings us closer. You can play with sharing secrets as a way to build intimacy with the section coming up.

Sharing our secrets, or any vulnerable information, means handing another person a way to hurt us, and when they don't use the information against us, that brings us closer. So when we're learning to talk to our partners, we also need to learn how to listen. We need to figure out how to hear what's being said fully, before we let our minds start racing with how that information affects us. We need to listen without planning how we're going to respond. And we need to listen with kindness and empathy. It's the only way to build strong and lasting relationships.

Read on for ways to practice not only communicating your needs, but valuable listening skills, too.

RELATIONSHIP BOUNDARIES

"The idea of choice in relationships is key in any relationship structure. Monogamy is considered automatic and the 'normal' way of being in a relationship. But I believe all relationships would benefit from actively choosing to be with one another within whatever relationship structure works for those particular partners."

—RENA MCDANIEL, *PRACTICAL AUDACITY*

3

Whether you choose to be monogamous or in some variety of open relationship, it's important to discuss the specifics of what that means to you. Many hurt feelings, and sometimes even breakups, happen because a relationship boundary was crossed that one party didn't even know existed.

Like with sex, we consider what we think about relationships to be obvious, and so we don't always voice our assumptions about what being in a relationship means. Sometimes we haven't even been explicit about *being* in a relationship.

Say you've been hanging out with someone for a while. You go on dates, you have sex, maybe you've even met some of each other's friends. These things often progress organically, such that a "let's talk about us" conversation never happens. In this scenario, it would be easy for one person to think that was a capital-R relationship, while the other person has another word for what they're doing, or maybe no word at all.

Say the person who thinks it's a relationship also thinks that relationships are always sexually exclusive, while the other person either doesn't think this is a relationship, or even if it is, they are used to open relationships. They might have sex with someone else, truly believing there's no reason not to. But when the person they've been spending time with finds out, they could be crushed.

Things like this can happen without anyone acting maliciously. But even without cruel intentions, feelings can get hurt.

This is why it's always best to be absolutely explicit about any expectations you might have. If you've reached a point with someone where you expect them to be monogamous, that needs to be explicitly communicated. Not only that, but you need to define what monogamy means to you. You might be rolling your eyes at me right now, saying surely this one *is* obvious to everyone.

Not so fast.

What about going out for drinks with a coworker of the gender you're attracted to, just the two of you?

What about a quick kiss on the lips as a greeting with a close friend? Or with a former partner?

What about talking about your sex life with friends? Or with strangers on the Internet?

What about watching porn, reading erotica, or masturbating?

Each of these are examples I've heard that led to fights because one person thought the activity was clearly innocuous, while the other thought it was a breach of their monogamy.

And these are just a handful of examples. I'm sure you can think of a lot more. And, in fact, I encourage you to.

As an exercise, sit down and think about what being in a relationship means to you. What do you consider fidelity, or loyalty? What emotional or sexual boundaries do you expect to maintain in a partnership?

Also, it can be helpful to think about which of those are absolutes that you need in place for your own well-being, and which could be negotiable. Sometimes you won't know this until it comes up, but it's useful to know where there's room for healthy compromise.

Here are a few things you can think about:

▸ Flirting
▸ Hugging
▸ Kissing
▸ Cuddling
▸ Holding hands
▸ Seeing someone naked in person (strip club, sex club, etc.)
▸ Seeing people naked online (webcams, etc.)
▸ Exchanging pictures online/by text
▸ Sharing fantasies or dirty talk online
▸ Seeing certain TV shows or movies with someone else
▸ Going to special restaurants, parks, or other significant locations
▸ Having a crush on someone else
▸ Falling in love with someone else
▸ Sleeping in the same bed with someone else (platonically)
▸ Sex with someone else, when out of town
▸ Going to sexy or kinky parties

Once you've gone through these ideas and added your own, compare lists with your partner. And make sure to drill down to specifics as much as possible. You can't think of everything that might come up, but having an open dialogue about these issues is really helpful.

Make sure this doesn't become about policing someone's behavior, but instead talking about each of your comfort levels with the different activities.

CROSSED BOUNDARIES

No matter how much talking you do, there's always a chance that a boundary will be crossed at some point. If that happens, have a conversation about *why* it happened. Was the boundary unclear or unknown? Was someone acting out because they don't think the boundary is fair? Only by figuring out *why* it happened can you address the real problem.

If an apology needs to be made, read on to learn how to apologize effectively.

HEALTHY BOUNDARIES VS. CONTROL

Talk of boundaries can get complicated, fast. Especially in open relationship circles, there are a lot of differing ideas about how to express boundaries in a relationship. Some people who practice open relationships are very couple-centric, or hierarchical. For these folks, it's very common to have explicit rules about what can and can't happen with other people, sometimes with a great degree of detail.

For other people, like relationship anarchists, these boundaries sound like coercion or unhealthy levels of control and are considered unfair both to the partner and to the additional people that person might engage with.

The minutiae of these distinctions are beyond the scope of this book, but it is valuable to take a look at some of the broader issues around establishing boundaries so you can make an informed decision when you're considering your own boundaries.

Before you establish any boundaries, think about why you want them and how they'll affect your relationship. We often set rules (and call them boundaries) to help manage our own fears or insecurities. In these cases, it can be helpful to work on our own feelings and responses rather than trying to control our surroundings and relationships. Because ultimately, not everything can be controlled, and we'll have to confront those feelings eventually.

Boundaries are about taking care of ourselves. Every time you feel uncomfortable or upset, it's a chance to learn something about yourself, and perhaps to learn about a boundary you need to set.

If you're dating someone who likes to be spontaneous and make last-minute plans, and you're someone who likes to know your whole week's schedule in advance, that can be a problem. Perhaps this person says to you, "Maybe we can get together on Friday?" And you agree and put Friday in your calendar. Then Friday rolls around and you don't hear from them. You text, only to find out that they ended up going on a weekend trip. They thought the plans were tentative; you didn't. If this upsets you, you might need to set a boundary about scheduling. Maybe you tell people you're involved with that you plan a week in advance, and if they want to see you, they need to plan in advance, too.

That won't work for some people, and that's okay. We always have to filter for folks who are a good fit for us. Doesn't mean the spontaneous person or the schedule-oriented person is wrong—they just might not be right for each other. But maybe scheduling a date night is no big deal for the spontaneous partner and they're happy to do it in order to see you. Then that person knows what you need, and that clarity can set people at ease. And you can feel calm about your schedule rather than resentful as you wait by your phone for them to call.

Saying what kind of notice you need for scheduling a date is ultimately about you. But things tip over into being controlling when you're making rules about what a partner can do or how they can use their time. If instead of saying you needed notice for dates, you said, "You can't take that weekend trip with your friends because I'll be lonely without you," that isn't a boundary anymore, that's exerting control. Controlling behavior often works to isolate people from their friends and family, and is one of the red flags to look out for in an abusive relationship.

"Controlling behavior can start small, such as dictating someone's schedule or whereabouts, but can morph into abusive dynamics when the power imbalance increases. Some of the signs of this include the use of manipulation, coercion, threats, or verbal or physical harm to enforce the power imbalance. Every member of a relationship must have the right to give feedback, seek compromise, set personal boundaries, and express thoughts and feelings safely. One of the reasons we seek to exert control is as a way of managing anxiety, insecurity, fear, or loss. When we can identify those underlying feelings or needs we can be more effective in communicating boundaries, wants and needs with our partners. This can prevent us from using other tactics that can cause harm to our partner and the relationship as a whole. Someone's love for you, or commitment to you, does not preclude them from engaging in abusive behaviors to get their needs met. Likewise, your love for them does not mean you must accept these patterns to get your needs met. If you're worried you're experiencing these dynamics and feeling unable to safely shift it on

> *your own, it's important to get help from a trained*
> *professional."*
>
> —ANGIE GUNN, LCSW CST

Most of all, trust your gut. And if something doesn't feel right, run it by a friend, family member, or therapist. The desire to please a partner can be very compelling, so make sure you check in with yourself on a regular basis to see how you're feeling about your relationship.

If you need more information about how to recognize abusive relationships, check out RAINN (https://www.rainn.org) and the Domestic Violence Taskforce (http://www.4vawa.org/get-help/).

EXPECTATIONS

One of the quickest ways we get into trouble is by expecting our partners to read our minds. The problem is, we don't always know we're doing it. It's natural to assume other people feel the same way we do about things. You've heard the adage "the problem with common sense is that it's not common"?

That happens to us in relationships, too. Whether it's how you think sex should go ("I perform oral sex on you and then you perform oral sex on me") or sharing household chores ("I cooked, so you do the dishes"), just because something seems perfectly clear to you doesn't mean the other person is on the same page.

Sometimes it's hard to figure out our expectations in the abstract. One surefire way to figure out when an expectation isn't being met? When you're feeling upset or frustrated. When that happens, it's important to think about why it happened. Were you expecting to hear from your partner and they never called? Did you think if you gave them a massage, they'd offer you one in return?

Often it turns out we had an expectation we never articulated. These examples have easy fixes: tell your partner what you want. It could be, "I'm going to have a stressful day, so can we have a phone call in the evening?" Or "My back is killing me, would you like to exchange massages?" It's important that we give our partners a chance to meet our needs before getting upset that they haven't magically done it.

If this is new for you, it might be tricky at first, but try to articulate as many of your expectations as possible to your partner. That way they can agree to meet those expectations, or they can negotiate something different. But you're not stuck with emotional land mines when unspoken expectations aren't being met.

In the example of someone not calling, say you practiced the ask, that you were having a bad day and would like to talk. Your partner could say, "Actually, I have a meeting that's running late and then I need to get to the airport. Could you hang out with a friend tonight and I'll call you in the morning?" That way you have a heads-up that they can't meet your exact request, and you have a chance to make a backup plan to get your needs met.

To avoid hurt feelings and miscommunications, it's a great idea to sit down and figure out what all of your assumptions and expectations are. You can do this alone first, and then have a conversation with your partner about it. For starters, see if you can make a list of absolutely everything you expect.

When you're making your list, here are some things to think about:

▸ Hygiene
▸ Household chores
▸ Communication frequency (daily, etc.)
▸ Reciprocity of sex acts
▸ Talking about feelings
▸ Saving a TV show that you started together for a time when you're together
▸ Friday or Saturday as a reserved date night
▸ Checking in on stressful/big days
▸ Sharing big life news
▸ Expectations around holidays or birthdays

Holidays and birthdays are one of the areas we most often expect mind reading. Many people think being in a capital-R relationship means holidays together are obvious, but as we're learning, nothing is obvious. Instead, make sure you're explicit about expectations when it comes to these events.

Do you want a present from your partner/lover for your birthday? Say so! Maybe it sounds strange to you to ask for a present, but not everyone is on the same page around this kind of thing.

Think about the love languages, a book and online quiz that help distill and discuss what kind of behaviors, activities, and words make us feel most cared for. For some people giving/receiving gifts is huge. For others, it's all about quality time together. So it would be totally reasonable for one person in a couple to expect a birthday present while the other person took a day off work or planned a special day together. Neither person is in the wrong—they just had mismatched expectations.

That's why it's important to talk about everything, even the things we think are obvious. Because what's obvious to us isn't always obvious to other people.

For me, it's important to get a wrapped present on my birthday from my intimate partner(s). It's not about the monetary value of the gift; it's about someone taking the time to acknowledge my birthday in that way. To me it speaks of thoughtfulness.

So when I was partnered to someone who said they weren't good at gift giving, we worked out an explicit agreement. I made it clear that a wrapped present on the day of my birthday was important to me, but to make things easier on them I'd send a wish list (with direct links to items) well in advance.

Sure, it took away some of the aspects of gift giving that I enjoy—having evidence that the person knows what kind of things I like—but it was a better compromise than letting them get overwhelmed with the task while I was disappointed with the results.

SHARED GOALS

Whether it's domestic/nesting projects like a garden or a new paint job, or working toward running a marathon together, having a shared goal is a great way to build camaraderie and intimacy in a relationship.

Building and maintaining a sexual connection that meets everyone's needs is also a shared goal that can be a priority in a relationship. Prioritizing that connection can mean setting aside a certain amount of time for intimacy, or committing to trying and learning new hobbies or new ways to connect.

Treating it like an exciting, ongoing exploration is a wonderful way to prevent sexuality from getting stagnant, and to make enough space for experimentation with which you can find new things you enjoy. And this is another area where the journey is (at least) half the fun. We don't want to set goals that are difficult to meet. Instead, we want to make the process the goal.

So, if someone is ejaculating sooner than they'd like, they shouldn't frame it as "I want to last ten minutes before ejaculation." That's a goal that can lead to frustration and failure and might be unrealistic for their body. Instead, they could frame it like this: "Together we're going to find new ways to experience pleasure that don't involve penile penetration, so that how long it takes to ejaculate doesn't feel like a limit to the length of intimacy."

If you've never had an orgasm, don't say, "I'll have an orgasm by the end of the year." Instead try, "I'm going to find new ways to relax and feel present in my body, and new ways to experience arousal and pleasure both alone and with my partner." Not only are these goals where the process of meeting them is the point, but if they take the pressure off meeting a certain outcome, that outcome might come along for the ride, too.

Just like training for a marathon, you need to celebrate your wins along the way. Have steps or milestones identified in advance, so that you can feel good about making progress, rather than just looking toward a goal that seems miles—or years—away.

Need some suggestions for shared goals?

▸ Plan one sexual and one nonsexual adventure together.

▸ Learn a new sexual technique either from books, videos, or in-person classes.

▸ Have a lengthy sexual and intimate experience that never involves genital touch.

▸ Share three new fantasies with your partner.

▸ Have regular date nights (even if sometimes they're Netflix and popcorn).

▸ Engage in more nonsexual touch.

▸ Try changing up your usual roles.

▸ Find a new toy or lube to try together.

Once the ideas start flying, you're likely to come up with plenty of your own ideas. Just keep them positive and realistic, and make sure to celebrate along the way.

DELIBERATE CHOICES

One of the precedents you want to set is making deliberate choices about what's best for you (and the relationship) rather than following any false timelines. Relationship books and the Internet are full of advice about everything from when to have sex to when to move in together to when to get married. Not only does this harmfully assume there's only one trajectory for a relationship, but it also assumes there's a one-size-fits-all approach. But nothing could be further from the truth.

Trying to meet outside expectations, whether from friends, family, or the culture at large, is a surefire way to end up with regrets. We can play along with what other people want from us for so long.

Establishing open communication early on means you can talk about what's right for each of you rather than falling into preworn paths on the relationship escalator.[2]

This can start as early as when you're chatting with someone on dating apps. Whether you want to ask someone out during the first text volley or chat for a few weeks before meeting, you get to decide what's right for you. Your choices will weed out some people, but that's what you want. You can also explicitly let the other person know what works for you, either saying, "Hey, it's hard for me to get to know someone by text, why don't we just meet up for coffee?" or "It takes me a little while to feel safe before meeting, so I'd like to text for a while to get to know each other." Whichever path you choose, you're staying true to yourself and not pushing outside your comfort zone based on a prescribed timeline.

Doing this also sets the precedent that you stand up for the timelines and communication styles that work for you. So the next time you let someone know what you need, they'll understand that's part of how you take care of yourself.

LESSONS FROM NONMONOGAMY

Whatever relationship structure is right for you, there are lessons to be learned by the way other people do things. It can be helpful to pick up books about relationship structures you might not want to engage in yourself, just to see

---

2   Relationship Escalator: "The default set of societal expectations for intimate relationships. Partners follow a progressive set of steps, each with visible markers, toward a clear goal." https://offescalator.com/what-escalator/

if there are any principles you can apply to your own life. While nonmonogamy certainly isn't for everyone, there are some features of that relationship style that can be helpful no matter what kind of relationship you want to have.

One of the principles of nonmonogamy is that you can't get all your needs met by one person. And while with nonmonogamy the answer is often sex with or dating multiple people, the principle stands for other activities as well.

Hoping for one person to meet all your needs for support, comfort, and entertainment is unrealistic. Sometimes, there are times when processing with your partner isn't the right choice, so having a strong network of friends you can talk to is essential. But all too often people can fall into a happy relationship bubble, especially early on in the romance, and can end up neglecting their other connections. When that happens and then you hit a rough patch, you may realize you don't have as many people to reach out to as you once did.

It's also important to have your own hobbies and interests. Whatever those activities are, it's healthy to have some time doing your own thing, apart from your partner. Not only is this independence an important reminder to yourself that you stand on your own two feet, but if you never did anything separately, what would you talk about?

This is a rut some long-term couples fall into. Their social lives are all together, and so they both already have all the same information. But when you engage in your own hobbies and activities, you can come home and share stories, and share things you're excited about. This makes us healthier individuals and more interesting partners.

Another concept from nonmonogamy that can serve

everyone is compersion. In the simplest terms, compersion is the word for feeling happy for your partner's happiness. Although in polyamory this most often applies to their happiness with other partners, it can just as easily apply to their happiness spending time with friends, or enjoying their work, or participating in other activities.

Our culture tells us we're supposed to spend every moment together, so it can be easy to get jealous not only about flirting or dating, but about activities that don't include us. If you work toward feeling a sense of compersion, it can get easier to understand that we all need a range of people and activities to fulfill us, and our partner's working on their own happiness benefits us as well.

Another lesson that folks in open relationships have to learn that can benefit everyone is an ability to embrace change and growth. I get it. Change can be scary. It's also unavoidable, and good for you! None of us stays the same over our lifetimes, and that's a good thing. So whether it's relationship needs shifting, or sexual interests shifting, or even a change in careers, it's important to be able to roll with change so that your relationship isn't derailed every time change is in the air.

The fear is often that if our partners change, there won't be room for us in their lives anymore. And it's true—sometimes people grow and change in ways that make the existing relationship no longer possible. But resisting that change by stifling your partner's ability to grow or evolve isn't any better. Not only is that unhealthy, but it's even more likely to end a relationship. The best course is for everyone in a relationship to keep working on themselves and making the choices that are best for their own personal growth. In this way, even if your paths are slightly different, you can keep supporting each other's progress.

TALK EARLY, TALK OFTEN: SEX

"Not asking for what you want in bed because you don't want to 'kill the moment' is like keeping plastic on the furniture because you want to 'keep it nice.' "

—JOELLEN NOTTE

I love talking about sex. I also love talking during sex. I love hearing what my partners want and how they feel. And I've learned that giving some guidance and feedback is also the best way to get the most pleasure for myself. But I understand that this is daunting for a lot of people.

I think one of the reasons people think it "ruins the mood" to talk or check in during sex is because they think of talking that would break a long silence. Maybe even hours of silence.

Sure, if you kiss on the front steps and then pull someone into your house, make out on the couch for a while, remove clothes, move into the bedroom, and then after all those assumptions and all that silence, begin detailing how you like to be touched, it might feel a little awkward.

So set the precedent for open communication right from the beginning. Ask before you kiss—maybe even before you step close to the other person. This can be incredibly sexy, as well as setting the other person at ease. Then ask if they'd like to come inside.

Once you're on the couch, have a negotiation about what will happen that evening, and have your safer-sex talk if you haven't done that already. Then check in before moving to the bedroom.

This way, by the time you need to give guidance, talking will be a well-established part of your interaction, and it won't have to be scary or awkward.

Here's one way that could go:

Sonya and Mitte have had a lovely date. Dinner is followed by a walk along the waterfront, and their conversation is going so smoothly it feels like they've known each other forever. They stop to watch a passing boat, and Sonya asks, "May I stand closer to you?"

Mitte tingles at the thought of Sonya in her personal space and says, "Yes," while also stepping closer to close some of the distance herself. They watch the boat together, close enough that their arms are brushing against each other, but before long they're watching each other.

"I love the way your hair frames your face. May I touch it?" Sonya asks, and Mitte gets chills again at the mere thought of the contact.

"Yes," she says, and then Sonya's hand is there, feeling the softness of Mitte's hair and pushing it behind her ear. Her hand lingers for a moment, and Sonya can see the goose bumps her touch has caused.

"I'd love to kiss you, would that be okay?" Sonya asks, and this time Mitte just nods and tilts her face up to be kissed without answering in words. They kiss, and it's slow at first as they get used to the feel of each other's lips. The kiss lingers, as their mouths explore, and Mitte's tongue darts out to taste Sonya's mouth.

After a few moments they part and just look at each

other until Sonya blushes and drops her eyes. "Shall we walk?" she asks, trying to mask her sudden shyness.

"Yes, let's," Mitte answers, and adds, "Can we hold hands?"

Sonya takes her hand, and they continue to stroll together, taking in the view.

You can see how in this interaction, the questions asked are part of the flirting and foreplay and don't ruin the mood at all. You can also imagine that if these two went home together, it would be part of the already established flow to ask for permission before doing something new, and to communicate about what they want.

Play around with it and find a style of communication that fits your personality. For some, playful banter is a good fit. For others it's being clear and direct. Some might even be shy, and say so, and express their needs while blushing. Whatever works for you is fine, as long as you're able to speak up for your needs and boundaries, and able to check in with your partner about theirs.

TALK EARLY, TALK OFTEN: RELATIONSHIPS

It's a lot easier to set a good precedent early on than to change things up once you have well-established routines. This can cover everything from boundaries to scheduling to ways of communicating.

Within what we're calling "good" communication, there can be many different communication styles. If someone doesn't communicate in a way that works for you, or in a way that's compatible with your communication style, it doesn't automatically make them a bad communicator. You might just have incompatible communication styles.

Some people like to talk things through, at length, whenever something comes up. Other people are considerably less verbose. While a certain amount of communication is absolutely necessary for a relationship, there are still many places on the communication spectrum where people can fall. That doesn't mean either person is doing it wrong, but it could mean they aren't a great fit for each other.

You can start feeling out someone's communication style early on. If when you're first texting with someone they take days to respond each time you reach out, this is a clue to their communication style. Too many people think that when something becomes a "real" relationship, everything changes. But nothing just changes by magic. If you expect to hear back from someone right away, or within the same day, you need to say so. Don't wait until you've been talking for weeks or months. If the communication style isn't working for you, say so. It'll only be harder once you're more invested, because the deeper we get into relationships, the more likely we are to let the "little things" go. But those things can add up. And you don't want to have bitterness building up over time.

To talk about what you need in relationships, you have to know what you need. It's worth taking some time to think about what's important to you. You can think about past relationships and make notes and lists about what was great and what needed work. From this, you can start to figure out your must-haves and your deal breakers.

Getting what we need is a combination of filtering for who is able to meet your needs when you're dating and communicating your needs to people once you get involved. There's no one way to be in a relationship, and expecting that people will just know the relationship "rules" gets people into all kinds of trouble.

Pay special attention to all of the assumptions we unpack later in this book and try to list and articulate all the wants and needs you have in relationships.

When it comes to anything to do with sex or relationships, you can't just have one conversation and be done with it. People change, situations change, and issues will always come up. So it's helpful to understand that many things will be a work in progress, that you may address more than one time.

This also means that when you're having a difficult conversation, sometimes it can be helpful to table the issue for a few hours or days, so you can either take time apart to cool off or focus on time together to rebuild connection before returning to the discussion when both of you are feeling able to be present and at your best again.

SOMETIMES IT'S UNCOMFORTABLE

Making change is uncomfortable.. Whether it's starting a new routine at the gym or learning a new skill, it takes a commitment of time and dealing with the fact that you won't be good at the new thing right away. And that can feel really hard. Especially when there's someone else around to see your learning curve.

But if you really want to have the best sex possible, you're going to have to come to terms with feeling uncomfortable or awkward sometimes. Not only is learning sexual communication learning a new language, but it's shifting lifelong, ingrained patterns.

The actual talking can feel uncomfortable, too. From conversations that are difficult to have to bodies doing things that are embarrassing or silly, there's simply no way to avoid being uncomfortable sometimes.

The trick is learning to embrace it. The same way you might appreciate the way your muscles feel sore after a workout, you can appreciate the process of learning new things with sex and communication. And if you're sharing this journey with a partner, the two of you can laugh about your missteps and awkwardness together.

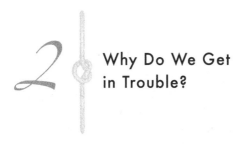

Why Do We Get in Trouble?

WE'RE NEVER TAUGHT THIS STUFF

SEX IS PERHAPS THE MOST COMPLEX ACTIVITY THAT we're expected to know how to do without ever being taught. Or at least without being taught well. Not only is good information generally missing from school curricula, but we're surrounded by misinformation.

My generation had stolen magazines and the occasional late-night movie. Younger folks have had the Internet—which is a mixed blessing in these areas.

Imagine being expected to sail, drive, or play chess without a book about it, without being shown by someone who already knows what they are doing, and without even being allowed to talk about it. That would never happen! The more complex or important the task, the more formal the training.

Maybe you heard adults whispering about the topic and then shushing their voices when you entered the room. Sex becomes the greatest mystery, but with so much shame surrounding the topic that you know not to ask without ever being told.

And thus, our problems are compounded. Not only are we not taught what to do—or how to talk about it—we're also raised with varying degrees of shame surrounding our bodies and all the things that bodies do.

Really, it's almost a miracle that anyone is having good sex.

And while we still have a very long way to go, there are now decent resources online, many fabulous books, and a new generation of sex shops that carry high-quality, body-safe toys, as well as offering a range of educational options.

Here in Portland, I'm lucky to have SheBop, a store with an amazing staff who give out valuable information about sex and bodies every single day. I also get to teach there, once or twice a month, along with a lineup of other incredible educators, and together we're bringing the idea that sex can be fun, safe, and pleasurable to more and more people.

The good news is that all these resources are available now, and you're already on the path to learn more. If this book leaves you hungry for more knowledge, check out the resources section in the back of this book and look for classes in your city.

A little knowledge goes a long way, and the more you can learn about sex, the more your own sex life will improve.

GAME PLAYING

Just about every rom-com would have you believe that if a partner can't read your mind, there's something wrong with them. Media shows examples of passive aggression, game playing, and impossible expectations. And because we're never taught healthy communication techniques, it's easy to see how some of these tactics become the norm.

Playing games isn't just a failure of communication, it's immature and will ultimately sabotage a relationship. Whole movies and TV series have been built around the idea of "testing" a partner, by putting them in manufactured situations and seeing how they perform. I'm a total social science nerd, and I'm all for doing your own research, but the main tenet of ethical research is informed consent—just like in relationships!

So don't pretend you're okay with going to a strip club or a sex club or having a threesome if you really aren't. You want your partner to be able to trust what you're telling them, not second-guess your real feelings and motivations.

We want to build trust in relationships, not undermine them. And this kind of game playing is guaranteed to teach your partner that they can't trust you with their real feelings and desires. And although pretending might work for a little while, it's ultimately unsustainable.

Instead of playing games, think about what you want to know and then find a direct way to ask. And when you do that, be ready for the real answers.

If you ask your partner if they think your best friend is attractive, and they say "yes," don't punish them for their answer. Thinking someone else is attractive doesn't mean they think you're any less attractive, or that they're thinking of cheating on you.

When you feel nervous about something—like your partner's attraction to other people—try to examine where that's coming from. Are you feeling insecure? Is it because your partner doesn't provide reassurance? Or maybe they compliment you all the time and you don't believe them? Usually when we're feeling uncomfortable, that's a sign that we have something we can learn about ourselves and our needs.

It's okay to directly ask for reassurances rather than trying to trick your partner into an answer you'll find reassuring. Try something like this: "I know you think my friend is attractive and I'm feeling insecure about that. It would help me to hear that you're attracted to me, or to hear something specific you like about my body." Most of the time our partners are thrilled to give us the reassurance we need, especially if it's asked from a place of honest vulnerability.

There's another kind of game playing we do that often stems from our own insecurities, and that's asking our partners questions that almost certainly require them to lie to us. The classic example we hear from stand-up comedians is, "Do I look fat in this dress?" Now, that question is also loaded with gender assumptions and stereotypes, but it hits a nerve. If you're looking for reassurances that back your partner into a corner, you may be forcing little white lies into your relationship.

And I don't know about you, but I want to be able to count on my partners, or the people I live with, to tell me the truth. If I'm getting ready for an event and I try on a dress that doesn't suit me, I want them to tell me! I don't want them to expect it's a trick question, which forces a lie, only to see pictures from the event later and realize I could have made a better choice.

We also force our partners into a difficult position

whenever we ask a question that compares us to other people, especially their past partners. Asking if you're the best sex they've ever had, or the best cook, or the prettiest, or if one of your body parts is the biggest, etc.

These questions can come from an understandable need for reassurance, but they're not the best questions to ask to get the reassurance you need. The fact is, someone is choosing to be with you. And the reasons we choose partners can be complex. Most of us aren't just shopping for the biggest penis, or the biggest boobs, or the person who can make the best lasagna. So comparing yourself on just one point doesn't really take in the whole picture.

Try questions like these instead: "Can you tell me something you enjoy about our sex life?" Or "Can you tell me what your favorite thing is about being with me?" Be sure to preface questions like this by saying you're feeling insecure, or that you'd like some reassurance.

WINNING

We're a competitive culture. We yell at sports games, we make bets, and we love being right. Just look at a winning team cheering at pub trivia. But don't let that impulse to win an argument or be right come before the relationship.

We've all been there, and I'm no exception. I remember being so invested in a partner learning the "right" way to load the dishwasher that it became a regular argument. Often, when things like dishes or laundry are a constant source of strife, it's an indication that other things are going on. For many people, there's an issue that's the canary in the coal mine of the relationship, whether that's underwear on the floor, or being on time to dates, or deciding which movie to see.

Things that might go mostly unnoticed when we're happy with a partner and with a relationship can become a much bigger deal when we're harboring larger concerns or irritations. So pay attention to what's getting under your skin, and if you catch yourself sweating the small stuff, take some time to see what's really going on.

The urge to win also comes up in the sexual arena. Sometimes people's desire to please their partner becomes competitive or ends up being about their own ego and not their partner's pleasure after all. If you're giving yourself a pat on the back for how many orgasms your partner is having with you, take a moment. Being an awesome lover can be a wonderful thing, but if it's more about the imaginary "best lover" trophy on your mantel than it is about your actual partner's enjoyment, then there can be a problem.

Our partners can tell when our motivations are complicated by ego, and that's one of the reasons people sometimes feel pressured to fake orgasms. But as soon as you're faking sexual pleasure for the sake of your partner's feelings, your chances of actual pleasure plummet.

We train our partners not just with verbal communication but with nonverbal communication. If we keep faking an orgasm when they do *that one move,* they'll think it really works for us. And that means they're likely stopping before a real orgasm is had. And it also gets harder to ask for what we really want if our partner thinks everything they're doing is blowing our mind.

You can still go yell at sports games if you want to, but try to keep the competition out of the bedroom.

FAIRNESS/SELFISHNESS

Our culture villainizes terms like *neediness* and *selfishness*. But it's vital to know what your needs are and to express them. There's no shame in having needs. We all have needs. And a lot of the time you *must* put yourself first. It's your job to get your needs met. However, the fear of being labeled needy or selfish often keeps us from asking for what we want from our partners.

One issue that's common is the idea of equality or parity of acts. For example, if one person loves receiving oral sex but their partner doesn't, the first person might be unwilling to ask for oral sex because they feel like they can't return the favor.

It's okay if your needs aren't exactly the same. They rarely will be. There can still be equity of time and attention paid to each other. In this example, maybe instead of oral sex the other person would love a foot rub or back rub or a different kind of sex act.

Here's the thing: if both people are looking out for their needs (and have the ability to say "no"), then it's always safe to ask for what you want. If you tell your partner you'd really love a back rub every day when you get home from work, they're free to agree to that, or to say, "I hear that you're tired and sore when you get home from work, but so am I. How about I aim for giving you a back rub once a week and we start saving up to get a couple's massage together?" As long as no is an acceptable answer (read up about requests vs. demands later) then it's safe to ask for what you want.

When all parties in a relationship stand up for both their needs and their boundaries, everybody wins.

YOU CAN'T GET WHAT YOU WANT IF YOU DON'T ASK FOR IT

When I'm working with clients, I'll often hear a long story about the things they'd like to try, or the needs they have, and hear their frustration with their partner. My follow-up question is always to ask whether they've told their partner the things they're telling me. Most of the time, the answer is no.

Imagine that. Telling me—often a complete stranger—their deepest desires is easier than telling their partner. That's really saying something. But there are few reasons why this happens.

For one, coming to my office means talking about sex. It's all over my website, in my writing, and hanging on the sign on my door. People know that talking to me about sex is safe. That's why they're there. They're confident I won't be judgmental. For the people who still aren't sure, they sometimes tiptoe around the issue. They'll check with me to see if discussing fetishes is okay. Or ask if they can use explicit language. (Yes and yes.)

But with me, the stakes are low. Sure, if they told me what they were into and I acted shocked, they might be embarrassed. But then they could leave and never see me again. If they tell their partner their desire and that person is shocked, well, the stakes are higher. People fear it could mean the end of the relationship, or at least a big, awkward elephant in the room for a while.

And that's understandable. Because anything even an inch out of mainstream sexuality (whatever that even means) becomes the butt of jokes everywhere from the locker room to late-night television. And people have an innate longing to fit in, so there's a chance you've laughed at those jokes, too. It doesn't even have to be mean-spirited. Some sexualities, kinks, or fetishes are presented as such a caricature that it's easy to forget that you're laughing at real people.

For all of these reasons, opening up about our interests can be terrifying. It can make people suppress their desires for years, even decades. But our sexuality is an integral part of who we are, and being able to express that sexuality is essential to our overall well-being.

Solving this problem is a team effort. We need to take responsibility for our own needs and desires and ask to get those needs met. *And* we have to make it safe for our partner to do the same.

How do you do that? For starters, you can tell your partner that you're a safe person to open up to. But you've also got to make sure that's true. Do your own work first by figuring out the biases you've acquired (that's coming up) and come to terms with everything that exists in the rainbow of sexual expression.

PERSONAL AND CULTURAL BIASES

Do you know where all of your beliefs about sex and sexuality came from? We're all influenced by the culture, society, community, and family we're raised in. If we want to start changing the kind of sex we're having with ourselves and with our partners, we'll need to unpack all our conscious and unconscious beliefs about sex and sexuality.

As you're reading about new kinds of sex you can try, you might feel a knee-jerk reaction that some things are wrong. Whenever that feeling pops up for you, take a moment to examine it and see if you can figure out where you first heard that message. Not only is this self-examination vital for your own sexual exploration, but it's important for making sure we don't unintentionally shame our partners with our responses to their sexual interests. So it's important to spend some time figuring out your biases, and all the things that make you uncomfortable, so you can process those reactions on your own before you end up hurting a partner's feelings.

The thing is, we don't always know what harmful baggage we're carrying around until something comes along to trigger it. And our beliefs are just that—beliefs. Until we're confronted with conflicting information, we can't know where we're wrong.

If you'd like to broaden your horizons when it comes to sex and sexuality, there are a few ways you can do that. A resource available for people training to become sex therapists or sex educators is called a SAR—Sexual Attitude Reassessment. They can vary a bit, depending on who is hosting, but the idea is the same. You spend a weekend learning about all different kinds of sex and kinks, often through seeing clips of porn.

As you watch different kinds of porn and listen to guest speakers, you're instructed to pay attention to the feelings and responses you're having to the content. The idea is to catch biases that you have, or things that make you uncomfortable, so you can examine those feelings in the space of the class. By going through this experience, you can be more likely to present a positive or neutral aspect when dealing with clients, rather than responding in a way that might shame them.

While I'm not necessarily suggesting you take the seminar (though it wouldn't be the worst idea) I do think you can and should do some of this work on your own. While the average person might not need to be as informed, or as neutral, as a sexuality professional, it's still helpful to be able to listen to our partners with an open mind.

In case you think these biases are a thing of the past, here are a few sentiments I've heard:

▸ Liking butt stuff means you're gay.
▸ Liking kink means you think "regular" sex is boring, or that you've been abused.
▸ Using a vibrator/sex toy makes you numb or ruins "real" sex.
▸ Only older men can have difficulty with erections.
▸ An erection is required for sex.
▸ Desire for sex is different based on gender.
▸ Using lube means a failure of arousal.
▸ If you need to stimulate yourself during sex to have an orgasm, there's something wrong with you, or with your partner.
▸ You're "supposed" to bleed the first time you have vaginal penetration.

Did you read any of those and think, "Hey, I thought that one was true"? Then you've got a good starting point for seeking out more sex-positive information. And even if none of these got you, there's still always a lot to learn. If you're inspired to get more informed, here are a few ways you can get started:

▸ Read books about sex and kink! Not all books are created equally, and unfortunately, some contain harmful misconceptions so screen them for sex positivity. Check the resources section of this book for suggestions.

▸ Watch porn! Yes, some porn has its own problems, but there's a growing body of sex-positive, body-positive porn out there. And you guessed it—there are suggestions in the resources section.

▸ Read blogs and articles written/posted by sex educators and sexuality professionals.

▸ Go to classes. Many sex shops have educational offerings, and other sexuality nonprofits often do as well. Check out what's happening in your town.

The other thing you can do without a single book or class is simply listen to your partner with an open mind. Ask them if you can ask questions. And believe their answers. We're all experts on our own sexuality, and when we feel safe, we can teach others about ourselves, too.

ASSUMING THERE'S A "NORMAL"

"How should this work?" and "How does this normally work?" are questions I hear weekly, if not daily. It's not surprising, because one of the ways we learn is by comparison. Forget how to tie your shoes? You look at what the kid next to you is doing.

But not only do we generally not watch other people having sex (more on that later), there are too many ways that sex and bodies can work for watching just one or two people to be enough, even if it were an option.

All bodies are different. All people are different. There's no way to emphasize that enough.

Are there certain ways that bodies fit together that you

can try? Absolutely. But you can't stop there. You need to know how to customize those acts for yourself, to get optimal (or any) pleasure out of them.

Speaking of questions I hear on a regular basis, "Is it normal to be into _____" is a daily one. From kinks to fetishes to interest in a variety of genders—interest in anything that doesn't show up in Hollywood romantic comedies leaves people wondering if there's something wrong with them.

Ultimately, "normal" isn't a useful concept when it comes to sex or bodies. And if you're asking yourself a question with *should* in it, I suggest you look into that more deeply, too.

Without knowing what you're into, I feel pretty confident saying, yes, you're okay. And you're probably not the only one with that interest, either. As long as everyone involved is a consenting adult, you're good to go. I can't count the number of clients I've had who simply needed to hear that the thing they were into was acceptable. That it didn't make them a freak or a pervert (unless you've happily reclaimed those words, as I have for myself).

For a long time I expected something truly rare or off-the-wall when someone was shy about telling me what they were into. But now I know that it'll be something I've heard before—and that I'll be able to point the person toward other people who are into the same thing.

That doesn't mean your kink will be for everyone. And if the thing you're into is a little more rare, it could be harder to find someone to share it with you. But the

Internet has done marvelous things for helping us find our people, and it can probably do the same for you.

WE DON'T KNOW WHAT WE WANT UNTIL WE AREN'T GETTING IT

Have you ever been hangry? It's that feeling where you've let yourself get so hungry that you're cranky/angry and you won't be productive, let alone decent company, until you get some food. It's such a common experience that memes expressing the feeling are all over the internet.

But if it sucks so much, why do we let it get that bad? Just have a snack! Because of course, it isn't always that easy.

From our schedules being so full that we're running around for hours without checking in with our bodies, to simple poor planning and not having food with us—and not wanting to get fast food—we forget to take care of ourselves for a variety of reasons.

It also happens, sometimes, because we didn't even realize we were hungry until it was too late. Sometimes the feeling needs to be extreme before it breaks to the surface and commands our attention.

The same happens with sex and relationships. We often don't know we're missing something, or realize how missing something is affecting us, until the feeling gets extreme.

I've had students and clients who've made it all the way to retirement age before realizing they've never had the kind of sex they want to have. And sometimes there can be years between having the realization and doing something about it.

While many of us are privileged to be able to feed ourselves when we're hungry, we also benefit from knowing how to meet that need. That's one we're taught from the very beginning. But with sex, even when we realize there's a problem, we might not know what to do about it, or where to go for help.

Here's how you can start realizing when there's a problem—when you start feeling the first hints of frustration that you aren't getting what you want, pay attention. Listen to your body and to your feelings. See if there are consistent times when the feeling crops up. What triggers it?

Use the food example as a starting point. When you're hungry, or planning for a meal, you start thinking about what you might want to have. You think about your favorite restaurants, or favorite recipes to make. You imagine yourself eating that food and see if it sounds good to you. And from there, you start to make a decision about what to have for dinner.

But as you may have noticed, the hungrier you are, the harder it can be to make that choice. When we get hungry enough, it's hard to think straight. Maybe we're so frustrated that nothing sounds good. Or maybe everything sounds good and we can't choose. That's why sometimes you start with a snack, and once that sinks in, you plan your real meal.

The same thing can work with sex. You can use the tools in the "what do you want" section of this book the same way you'd scroll through nearby restaurants or the pages of a cookbook. You can consider your various options the way you'd consider a recipe and decide if they sound good. And for some things, you can have a snack or a taste to see if something appeals to you.

Sometimes that's what you have to do—sate some of

the hunger so you can think straight. Even if it's sexual hunger. You can try getting back in touch with your own body before involving a partner, if that feels easier. You can get a new sex toy or try new tools for arousal. Sometimes that helps take the edge off.

If you're trying it with a partner, try reestablishing intimacy and connection so you have a solid base for trying new sexual adventures. Or return to what's worked with them in the past before you start trying new things. Engage in whatever self-care you can so that you're not sexually hangry as you begin to explore and have new adventures.

"WHATEVER YOU WANT"

I can't even begin to count the number of times a new partner has told me, "You can do whatever you want to me." I've experimented with different ways of answering. Sometimes I make it a joke and say that demonstrates a lack of imagination. Sometimes I give an example of something I'm almost sure they wouldn't like—and I'm kinky and creative, so I've got a lot of ideas at my disposal.

I think the reason people say this so often is that we assume that whatever we think is part of the "normal" sex repertoire is the same for everyone. We can't even fathom that someone else's standard sex is different from ours.

For one person, anal sex might be their usual go-to. For another person, anal play might be entirely unfathomable. But our worldview feels so obvious to us, it's hard to understand that someone else can have a completely different set of operating procedures.

This is why we need to spend time unpacking everything we think about sex, sexuality, and intimacy. And this can be a long process that brings up lots of feelings.

You can do this as an exercise right now. Take out a notebook, or open up a blank page on your computer or phone. Start making a list of what you expect to be included in a typical sexual encounter. Maybe what you'd have on your "yes" list the first time you sleep with a new partner.

Kissing? Hand sex? Oral sex? Vaginal penetration? Anal penetration? Sex toys? Kink play? Drill into the details of each of those, what they mean to you, and what they include. And then get in the habit of sharing what you'd like your encounters to include with your partners to make sure you avoid any unwelcome surprises.

THE PERFECT IS THE ENEMY OF THE GOOD

When I was redesigning my website, I was taking ages to get each piece of content to my web developer. Things like my "about" section would stump me for months. As much as I love writing, writing about myself is a whole different story. So with each new page we were tackling, I'd drag my feet for weeks and months, and eventually the project had taken most of a year.

One day I got a simple one-line email from the web developer. It read, "The perfect is the enemy of the good." And it worked. I sent her what I had ready and said, "Let's just go with it."

Most of us are perfectionists in at least some aspects of our lives. And that affects us in sex and relationships, too. I've had students and clients that have held off on certain kinds of sex (or on sex altogether) because they feared they lacked the skills to do it well. That can be a good impulse if you're wanting to do something risky, like an extreme form of kink play, but when it comes to something where no one can get hurt, sometimes just fumbling through it and exploring as you go is the best thing you can do.

I get it, I really do. I don't like being bad at things in public. Many of the skills I've cultivated over my life are those that can be practiced in private before anyone has to see them. When I was a kid taking piano lessons, my family had to endure it, but beyond them I could choose if and when to have an audience. With my writing I can fiddle with it as long as I want (deadlines notwithstanding) before I show it to the world.

But some things require a partner, so at least one person is going to have to watch you learn. I struggled with this when I was new to rope bondage. Not only did my play partner see where I was with my skill set, but the instructor and other students could see, too. It took me a while to get used to fumbling through and being bad for a while, and it's still not my favorite thing to do.

But if you wait until things are perfect, you might not ever get to do them, especially when those things require a partner.

So give yourself permission to be new, to be learning, and to be not quite perfect.

ASSUMPTIONS AND MIND READING

I'm sure you've heard all the little sayings about assumptions. It's a common warning because it's true—assumptions get us into all kinds of trouble. The same is true when we attempt mind reading. Usually you hear about not expecting your partner to read your mind (and that's true, too), but it goes both ways. When we make assumptions about our partner's thoughts, needs, or feelings, we're asking for trouble.

People omit information with the excuse "I thought you'd be mad" all the time. And sometimes the original issue wouldn't have been a problem, but now the lying is what they're angry about. Or we simply work ourselves up thinking our partner won't be into something, only to find out they totally are, or at least don't mind if we are.

Our minds are funny things. For many of us, we jump to the worst possible outcomes in our heads and never let our partners actually let us know what is and isn't a big deal for them.

Like I keep emphasizing, one of the main ways we get into trouble is by having a set of assumptions that feel so commonsense to us, we don't even realize we have them. If we think something is obvious, we probably aren't saying it out loud. So what happens when an intimate partner has a different set of assumptions, or if their obvious doesn't match yours?

Well, that's when miscommunications happen that can range from something to laugh about together to hurt feelings or even tears.

You've heard the joke about the fish not knowing what water is? Well, that's how we are with our assumptions. So it takes some unpacking, and some trial and error, to figure out all the assumptions we're walking around with.

We can also get into lots of trouble assuming we know what a partner wants from a sexual or kinky encounter.

We're so prone to comparison that it's easy to hear a partner's stories of their past encounters and assume that's what they want from us. But what if what they like about us is the very fact that we're different? Launching into a kind of sex we assume they want can go sideways very quickly. It can blow past boundaries and even consent, and potentially reopen past traumas.

There's no way to know that what someone has liked in the past is what they'll like now. People change from day to day and year to year. The only surefire way to know what someone wants is to ask them.

On the romance and relationship side, assumptions are still problematic. Thinking about love languages can help you understand that different people have different ways of feeling appreciated and cared for. Whether or not you take the official quiz (and not everyone falls neatly into one category), it's helpful to know what makes your partner feel loved.

Maybe you want to do something nice for your partner, so you bring home a bouquet of flowers. Their first thought might be of the mess the flowers are going to make as they die. Maybe what would have made them really happy is if you took them out to dinner or cleaned the kitchen.

Like all other areas of relationships and sex, assumptions get us into trouble. There's no guarantee that what we like, or what a past partner liked, will work for our current partner.

WE DON'T BELIEVE PEOPLE

This comes up again and again—we don't believe people. I see it coming up with clients where one person doesn't believe their partner is enjoying sex. Maybe it's the media's portrayal of mind-blowing orgasms that contributes to this, but we seem to want some kind of proof that our partner is enjoying themselves. We want to see eye-rolled-back orgasms, or visible ejaculations, or spasms of pleasure. Without that, we doubt their enjoyment.

But when someone tells you they don't like something? We tend to believe someone right away. If you're rubbing someone's shoulders and they say it hurts—it's too hard—you'd believe them and adjust what you're doing right away. But if they assure you they're really enjoying the massage, we second-guess that. We think they're saying it to avoid hurting our feelings or because they're grateful they're getting a massage at all.

Do people ever say things for the sake of someone's ego? Sure. But the assumption that someone isn't telling the truth will cause far more trouble than the small percentage of exaggeration it'll weed out.

WE DON'T TELL THE TRUTH

On the flip side, if we want partners to believe us, we need to tell the truth. Whether it's faking orgasms, or saying you like giving or receiving oral sex when you really don't, lying about sex and pleasure undermines all sexual communication. And this includes lies of omission. If you engage in a sex act you're not enjoying, and you don't say anything about it, your partner will probably think it was okay, and is likely to do it again.

It's only going to get harder and harder to bring up, as time goes on, because your partner will almost certainly ask why it didn't come up sooner.

We want our partners to believe us, and to help

cultivate that trust, we need to be honest. Being honest about sex can feel scary, but it's the only way to get the kind of sex we want. Every time we lie about how much pleasure we're experiencing, or fail to say when something doesn't feel good, we're making it even harder to start having the kind of sex we will enjoy.

And it isn't just a matter of honesty around the sex we're having. Studies have shown that people lie to their partners about a wide range of topics relating to relationships and sexuality. It's hardly a surprise, given the sex-negative attitudes of our society at large. We've been trained to feel so much shame around topics relating to sex, and we've so often been backed into corners by family, church, and even partners that on some topics lying becomes second nature.

Wondering what topics are frequently the subject of dishonesty? Here are a few:

- ▸ Feelings for other people
- ▸ Contact with exes
- ▸ Porn use
- ▸ Masturbation
- ▸ Sexual fantasies
- ▸ Sexual history
- ▸ Sexual encounters with other people
- ▸ Satisfaction with current sex life
- ▸ Feeling insecure in the relationship

Whenever possible, start off on the right foot by being honest with a new partner from the very first encounter. From the first time their hand touches your body to the first time you kiss, get in the habit of giving feedback. If they touch you gently and you're ticklish, let them know you'd like a firmer touch. If they kiss with a lot of tongue and you'd like something less wet, ask if you can show them how you like to be kissed. Believe me, talking about these things is a lot easier than talking about more involved sex acts, so setting the precedent early will make it much easier when it comes time to talk about sex.

And beyond simply discussing sex, create an air of openness about all things relating to sex and sexuality. Rather than lying about watching porn, watch it together! Don't lie about masturbation—engage in mutual masturbation! Having a solid base of being able to talk about all of these topics will make it easier down the line when you want to talk about a touchy subject, like a new sexual fantasy you want to try or attraction to someone new.

If you've already been lying to your partner about pleasure, or at least not volunteering the truth, check out the section in Difficult Conversations below about how to start repairing that damage.

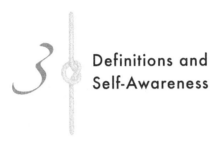

Definitions and Self-Awareness

WHY DO YOU WANT IT?

THIS BOOK WILL ASK A LOT OF QUESTIONS THAT you might think are silly—because you think the answer is obvious. But one of the main things I'm trying to unpack with this book is that what we think is obvious often isn't clear to others at all.

One of those questions is, why do you want to have sex? Pause and think about that a little. Think about why you desire sex in general and brainstorm your answers.

Once you've made your own list, here are a few more motivations to consider:

- Physical pleasure
- Orgasmic release for relaxation
- Orgasmic release for stress reduction
- Connection with your partner
- Expressing care or affection
- Expressing attraction or desire

‣ A desire to show off your own sexual skills
‣ Procreation
‣ Curiosity
‣ A sense of obligation
‣ Novelty
‣ Spiritual experience
‣ Boosting self-esteem

This list is far from exhaustive. A study reported in the *Archives of Sexual Behavior* identified 237 reasons people might have sex.[3] But for the sake of this exercise, it's enough to get you thinking and realizing there are more motivations than you might have consciously considered.

Now that you've thought more broadly about reasons for having sex in general, think about specific instances. Maybe you had sex to reconnect with a partner after one of you was away or had makeup sex after a fight. In these instances, it's often the intimacy and connection we're seeking.

Why are we doing this work? Because when you know what underlying need you're trying to meet, you can figure out if there are other ways to address that need. For example, if what you want is an orgasm to relax before bed and your partner doesn't feel like having sex, then maybe you can meet that need with masturbation. Maybe your partner joins in by watching porn with you, or snuggling with you, or maybe you're in separate rooms.

If what you're looking for is connection after being away, what are other things you could do to feel

---

3   Cindy M. Meston, David M. Buss, "Why Humans Have Sex," *Archives of Sexual Behavior* 36, no. 4 (2007): 477–507, https://doi.org/10.1007/s10508-007-9175-2.

connected? Maybe snuggling and talking about your trip? Or watching a movie while cuddling on the couch?

Here's the formula so you can try it yourself:

What needs are you trying to meet?

Is there another way to get that need met?

It can also be really useful to have this conversation with your partner. Even when you're both game for sex, you can still have different needs in mind. One person focusing on connection while the other is focusing on orgasm is still a potential mismatch. The only way to make sure everyone is getting their needs met is to be explicit about what they are.

This is what we're striving for in our sexual communication. Not just clarity in what we're saying, but clarity of intentions. Language is an imperfect medium, and no matter how hard we try there are going to be occasional miscommunications. But we can try to weed out as many places as possible where we're unclear.

WHAT ARE YOU ASKING FOR WHEN YOU SAY "SEX"?

A few years ago, I was hired to work a New Year's Eve party for a sex-positive organization. The party was being held in a three-story building, and each story had a different theme and a different level of sex play. I was working the dungeon level in the basement. My job was to teach and demonstrate a variety of kink toys and forms of play, as well as to supervise the people playing.

In order to do my job well, I needed to understand the party rules. I asked the host what was and wasn't allowed on this floor. They told me that nudity, along with kink and sexy play, was allowed, but no sex. I continued looking at them, expecting additional information, but it became clear they were done. So I asked, "What do you mean by sex?" They seemed confused by the question, and eventually answered, "Penetration."

Not wanting to be difficult, but also knowing I couldn't enforce rules if I didn't understand them, I had to continue asking questions. "What about penetration with fingers or toys?" The host stared at me blankly. They hadn't thought about this. Ultimately the organizers had to run off to have a meeting to define their terms before coming back to me with more clarity about what was and wasn't allowed. Well, if people running sex parties don't have a working definition of sex, it's no surprise that the average person dating or having relationships runs into trouble.

First you need to have an idea of what options are available, and what your own definition is. Then you can work on communicating that to others. When you're about to have sex with someone new, it's important to define what you mean by "sex" and what the scope of activities is going to be. This prevents all kinds of misunderstandings—from the uncomfortable to the dangerous.

Even in long-term relationships, it can still be important to check in about your definitions now and then. This can be an item for your state-of-the-relationship talk (more on that later). "Having sex" can become shorthand for a particular routine you've gotten used to. And if one or both people are tired of this routine, they might start saying no to sex. But it's very possible that a reworking of what sex means, and what it looks like, can make for more frequent, and better, sex.

When I was married, my spouse and I weren't always sexually compatible. And I didn't have the tools then that I do now to work on it. But this was one trick I did figure out from that situation. When he would ask for sex, I'd learned what he meant: he wanted to penetrate me until he had an orgasm. Typically he'd fall asleep after. There wasn't much in it for me, aside from some nominal connection.

So one day I told him the reason I often turned down sex was because I wasn't keen on what he meant by that. He was open to feedback, so I suggested he instead ask if he could give me an orgasm, or even a massage. I was far more likely to say yes to intimate contact if I knew I was going to get pleasure out of it. And nine times out of ten, once he'd done something like that for me, I was perfectly happy to reciprocate.

But if I'd never made the connection that there was as much a communication problem as a sexual problem, I might not have found a solution so easily. And our relationship would likely have deteriorated much more quickly. Although I can't promise that all sexual issues will be resolved so smoothly, getting on the same page about language is a huge step in the right direction.

REDEFINING SEX AND INTIMACY

It's no surprise we have a difficult time defining sex. Or at least a limited definition. The mainstream view of sex is pretty narrow. It tends to focus on penetration, generally by a penis into a vagina. This narrow view leaves a lot of people out in the cold. Not only is it a very cisgendered, heterosexual notion of sex, but it ignores people with different tastes or preferences, or people whose bodies work in different ways.

When we ask for sex, or when our partner thinks we

want sex, there can be an assumption that this narrow definition of sex is what's meant. Regardless of what genders or genitals are involved, many couples have a standard routine. And whatever your go-to sex looks like, that's what our partners are going to assume we mean. This can lead to a no when there might actually be room to find something that will make both people happy. So the wider a definition of sex and intimacy you have, the more likely you are to find activities two (or more) people can agree on.

What if genital touch wasn't required for intimacy, or even sex? What if your definition expanded to include bathing together, massaging each other, or even slowly cooking and savoring a meal together? You can get as creative as you like, from partnered yoga to rope bondage—there are lots of ways to engage with another person's body that can be done without genital touch, and even with clothes on.

Not only is our view of sex narrow, it tends to be goal oriented, with the usual goal being (mutual) orgasm. So what happens if one, or both, people don't easily reach orgasm? Does that mean sex and intimacy are off the table whenever their bodies aren't behaving exactly the way they'd like?

Tying into the problem of not believing each other about pleasure, if the body isn't demonstrating what we've come to expect as visible signs of arousal and enjoyment (like erections and lubrication) we doubt that our partner is enjoying themselves.

So if we know our body won't do what our partner is expecting, and we know we won't reach orgasm, it can be difficult to engage in activities that might still bring pleasure. Many people don't realize that massaging a vulva, or an anus, or touching a flaccid penis, can all still feel very good, even if there isn't an orgasm.

We also need to understand that using sex toys doesn't indicate some kind of failing, or cop-out, but instead is as basic as any tool we'd use for a job. When was the last time you heard someone being ashamed or embarrassed about using a hammer instead of pounding a nail with their bare hand?

Start thinking of intimacy, and even sex, as any activity you can do alone, or with a partner, that allows you to feel pleasure. And if you're not willing to go quite that far with me, how about this: Instead of thinking of sex that doesn't tick all the boxes you'd hoped as a failure, how about thinking of it as successful intimacy instead?

Maybe for you a massage, or any of the other suggestions I've made, just doesn't resonate with you as sex. That's fine. Instead, you can go into activities with a range of possible outcomes in mind. Perhaps you'd like to have penetrative sex, but if that can't happen, or it doesn't go exactly the way you'd hoped, you can still have a powerful experience of intimacy with your partner.

SPECIFICITY

One of the most common sources of miscommunication is a lack of specificity. We speak in vague terms so often, we don't always realize we're doing it. Imagine you're making a date and you ask if the other person wants to meet later that night. "Later" for one person could mean seven P.M. while for the other it means ten P.M. The two people could think they've come to an understanding, but when seven o'clock comes and goes, there could be anything from confusion to hurt feelings.

This can be even more dangerous when you're talking about sex or kink. The riskier the behavior (physically or emotionally), the more sure you want to be that you define your terms. If for one person spanking means gentle love taps during sex, and to the other it means hard swats with a paddle or belt, that's a discrepancy that can cause a lot of problems.

So what do you do about it? Well, if someone asks you if you're interested in trying something, ask for more information before you give an answer. Asking things like, "What does that mean to you?" can be a great way to clarify. You could also let them know what you think it means, and give them a chance to correct you, or fill in any missed details.

It's no wonder we run into problems when specificity matters, because the way we use our language colloquially, we often say the opposite of what we mean, in an attempt at humor, sarcasm, or emphasis. We say, "I'm a bit peckish" when we haven't eaten all day. We say "literally" when we mean figuratively. We say something was freezing, or on fire, when it was just a bit warm or cold for comfort. It's so ingrained in the way we speak, you might not even notice you're doing it.

So what happens if you keep that habit when talking about a delicate subject with a partner? Well, if you use your typical exaggeration and say, "I hate that thing you do," when really it just bothers you a little bit, you've probably just hurt your partner's feelings when you could easily have been more clear, or more specific, about what you mean.

If you're the one proposing something, head off confusion and misunderstanding by painting as clear a picture as you can, right from the get-go. Rather than saying, "Would you like to try some kinky stuff?" ask, "How would you feel about bending over my lap to get spanked with my hairbrush?"

"Kinky stuff" could mean just about anything, and if you leave the question at that, the other person's mind could be reeling with possibilities, several of which they may not be interested in. Get used to being specific with your requests, because then you can both be on the same page for negotiation. Rather than spending twenty minutes defining what "kinky stuff" means, you can spend that negotiating time discussing which hairbrush to use and how hard to hit with it.

CLARITY

The cousin to specificity is clarity. If you want to ask someone out on a date, say so. Sure, "Let's get coffee sometime" might be easier to force out of your mouth, but that leaves the other person wondering what you mean. Is it a friends thing? Professional networking? Something romantic? You don't want to get a yes only to find out at the end that they were there to get introduced to your marketing buddies.

Clarity is also very important when discussing sex acts. And I've had a couple interesting run-ins when it comes to getting clarity, or assuming something was clear when it wasn't.

On a date with someone, we were discussing our sexual histories and interests. They told me they'd tried anal sex a few times but weren't really into it. My immediate reaction was to ask a clarifying question—did they mean giving or receiving anal sex? They were so shocked by my question I thought for a moment they might choke on their dinner. It had never even occurred to them that that statement could mean receiving, whereas I figured it was fifty-fifty what they meant.

Butt stuff is often an area where we lack clarity of communication (even when we think we're doing a great job!). I had another date where we had negotiated hand sex and I was playing with the other person's body. I asked if I could touch their anal area and they said yes. I performed external massage for a while and then asked how they felt about penetration. They said that was fine. So I pulled my hand away to get more lube. As soon as they saw me lubing up my finger they realized what I meant and said, "Oh! You mean me!" I'd thought that asking while touching their anus made my intentions clear, but it hadn't. Even in that context, I'd needed to ask, "How would you feel about receiving anal penetration right now?"

Maybe you think that sounds awkward or clunky. But it's a lot less awkward than penetrating someone who wasn't expecting it—and maybe didn't want it. In fact, that lack of clarity can quickly become a consent violation. So being clear what we're asking for, and agreeing to, is essential.

When I was speaking at Portland State University, they introduced me to a clever way they handle this issue. As I was speaking at the front of the room, someone stood at the back and held up a sign that said DEFINE YOUR TERMS whenever I used a sex or kink word that was obvious to me but not obvious to everyone.

This was a fantastic reminder to slow down and make

sure my own assumptions weren't getting in the way of my audience having a clear understanding of what I was talking about. And while I wouldn't necessarily suggest you have a sign made up, it can help to ask your partners to define their terms—and to look out for defining your own.

Clarity applies to feelings, too. We need to make sure we're being clear with what we're trying to express. Think of the statement "I haven't been having much sex lately." That could mean the person simply hasn't had the time or opportunity, or it could mean they haven't been interested. If their intention was to tell a partner that they're not feeling very sexy and likely won't want sex that night, this could backfire. Because that statement could just as easily be read as a bid for sex.

Just because a statement is clear to us, it doesn't mean a partner will get our meaning. If you're trying to express something important, it's a good idea to check whether your partner understands you.

Most people undercommunicate, so if you aim for what feels like too much communication, you're probably getting closer to what's needed.

MOVING THROUGH DIFFICULT FEELINGS

As you begin to explore the wide world of sex and intimacy, you're bound to hit on things that make you uncomfortable, from feelings of jealousy to things that challenge your understanding of relationship models. The more you explore, the more likely you are to discover things you aren't into, or that push your buttons. And that's great! Finding out what you don't like, or what challenges you, can be just as useful as figuring out what you do enjoy.

If there's something you're simply not turned on by,

that's fine. But if something felt threatening or challenging in some way, it can be helpful to figure out why you're reacting that way.

When enough time has passed to explore your feelings, do some self-reflection. Maybe this is by journaling or talking to a friend—whatever works for you when you're trying to process. See if you can figure out what caused the difficult feelings.

Sometimes the very process of talking or writing will help you figure out where the feelings are coming from, and sometimes you can dig deeper by asking yourself some questions. For example if you're feeling jealous, dig a little deeper. Jealousy is actually a category of feelings that could include anything from not wanting your partner to be engaging in that activity at all to feeling left out because they're not doing it with you to feeling insecure because you think another person might be better at something than you are.

DON'T YUCK ANYONE'S YUM

Have you seen the Ze Frank video about yucking people's yum? If not, it's well worth a Google search. It's also a vital concept as we talk about exploring our fantasies and desires.

When someone opens up about their sexual interests, they're making themselves vulnerable to you. And it's your responsibility to listen to them in a way that does no harm. You don't have to be into what they're into. You don't need to do the thing with them. But you do need to avoid shaming them, or embarrassing them, about their desires.

This isn't just about partners. If you're going to explore

any kind of public sex or kink play, it's vital that you're ready to see things you're not into—maybe even things that shock or upset you. But the people who are participating in the activity are not the people to process those feelings with—and certainly not while they're playing.

Voices carry in play spaces, and if you're talking about someone and making judgments about their body or their play, they might hear you. Not only that, but the person you're talking to, or other people around you, might be into the same thing and feel shamed.

Because here's the thing—just because you don't like something, it doesn't mean that thing is bad or gross. Surely at some point you've had this debate about favorite foods, or pineapple on pizza. The pro and con camps are vociferous and insistent, and it's an absurd argument. How can a flavor of food be objectively right or wrong, good or bad? We all get to choose our favorite candy at the movie theater (or sneak in a chopped apple—whatever floats your boat), but nobody is better or worse for those preferences.

And the same goes for sex and kink. You're going to see things that are somebody's pineapple on pizza, and whether you're into it or not, you just have to let them do their thing. And if you're not into it, you can simply move away from the activity you're having trouble with and go watch something else. Rather than shaming them, it's far more useful to examine why that activity feels challenging for you and to do some more research on the topic if you'd like to explore those feelings.

JOURNALING

One of the most frequent homework assignments I give clients is to start keeping a journal. This can be a fabulous tool for tracking how you're feeling over time, or to track your growth or self-exploration. Journaling can also be a great first pass at processing whatever you're feeling about your relationship(s) or your sex life, and if something comes up more than once, that can be an indication that it's time to talk to your partner about it.

Your journal can be as simple or as elaborate as you'd like. It can be notes on your computer or your phone, or a physical notebook you use for the purpose. You can color code or add sticky tabs, or you can simply write freehand. Use whatever tools and writing style feels the most comfortable.

When can journaling be useful?

Journal after dates, to work through your feelings about the person. Were there red flags? Were there things you were excited about? Questions you want to ask next time?

Journal after sex, or kink play, to keep track of what worked for you and what didn't. Keep track of your favorite parts so you can ask for them again, and the things you weren't crazy about so you can modify them in the future.

Journal when difficult feelings come up. When you're feeling anxious, or jealous, or insecure. See if you can track what happened to trigger these feelings. Can you find a pattern over time?

Part of why journaling is not just useful, but important, is because it's our job to know ourselves. We need to know what we want so we can express those desires to a partner. (And if this is a sticking point for you, don't worry—there are exercises for you coming up.)

It's also helpful for noticing patterns of feelings—like maybe every time your partner is late getting home from work you're mad at them and avoid talking to them for the evening. Without writing it down, maybe you wouldn't notice the trigger of them being late setting off your feelings. Once you know what the problem is, you can address it, maybe by asking them to give you a more realistic idea of when they'll be home, or to call when they're on their way. Whatever the solution, you need to know the problem before you can get there.

The act of writing things down can also help you get to the bottom of your feelings. Maybe you're feeling something you interpret as jealousy, but when you spend some time thinking, and writing, about what you're experiencing, you realize that you're actually just missing your partner when they're away.

Our feelings can be elusive sometimes, and we need to narrow down what we're experiencing before we can talk about it in a productive way.

KEEP IT POSITIVE

Studies have shown that a shockingly high percentage of self-talk is negative. This can be our internal voice, what we say to ourselves when we look in a mirror or pass by our reflection, and it can also be what we're saying out loud about ourselves to our partner(s) or friends.

I first learned about this in college, when I was working toward my sociology degree, but learning it in the classroom was nothing compared to seeing this happen in real life. One summer I got a job at a clothing store at the mall near my college to help me pay for summer term. I hadn't expected working in the mall to be fun, but the job ended up being grueling in ways I'd never anticipated.

Women would come into the store to try things on, and they'd often want my help in the fitting room. I'd be asked to do everything from help with zippers to get other sizes to simply offer my opinion on the outfits. As I was doing this work a pattern quickly emerged: nearly every woman I joined in the dressing room would say something negative about her body as she looked in the mirror. Sometimes they were saying it to me, but mostly I think they were saying it to themselves, just ignoring the fact that I was there. Service workers often pass as invisible.

Lots of people complained about their weight, but many folks had specific complaints, too. People worried about their arms, their thighs, their necks . . . no body part was safe from criticism. Many of these women called me into the dressing room when they were nearly naked, not seeming bothered about me seeing them undressed, but then laying into themselves with negativity.

I must have been nineteen at the time, and I certainly didn't have the tools and awareness I have now. In fact, had I been the customer, I might have been right there with them, wishing I could lose a few pounds in the hope it would make me look better in the fashions of the day.

I did what I could to uplift and reassure them, but I'm not sure it did much good. I'm not sure anyone was really listening to me, or that they were ready to hear it anyway. The emotional labor of that piece of the job was more exhausting than the eight hours on my feet or the mundanity of spending days in the mall. I couldn't get out of there fast enough when my three months were up.

But that experience has stayed with me. It brought home what my professors were saying about negative self-talk in a way I never would have believed simply from lectures and textbooks. And when I talk to clients and students about it now, they usually recognize this trend in themselves, too.

And it isn't limited by gender. Most of the shoppers we got in that store were ciswomen, but I know from other spaces, and what people have told me, that no gender is immune to this kind of body negativity. Far too many people are striving for something that seems just out of reach, or waiting for some change in their physical appearance before they'll do that thing they're excited about.

But you know what? Those physical changes won't make you feel any better if you don't also address the habit of beating yourself up. The five pounds you wanted to lose will become ten. Or the focus on your arms will shift to your thighs. There's always some goal you can put between where you are now and the things you're afraid of trying.

I know this from my own experience, too. When my marriage opened up and I joined the local kink scene, I was amazed to see people gleefully undressing to experience various sensations against their skin, from spanking to flogging to whipping.

I'd just spent a decade working in an office, and pencil skirts, supported by Spanx, were my uniform. I'd finally found a personal style I felt good in, and I liked the classic secretary look and hearing my heels clicking on the floor as I walked. Then I entered these spaces and realized how absurd it would be to have so many layers to peel off. Not to mention how unflattering it was to wiggle in and out of Spanx, or the marks they'd leave on my body.

But as I looked around I saw that not everyone looked like a supermodel. These were real people, of a range of ages, genders, and body types, all enjoying how their bodies could *feel,* no matter how they *looked.*

The next party I went to I simply wore a slip that I could drop in a matter of seconds, and this time I tried all kinds of things I'd been curious about for years. And when I was up on the cross feeling a range of sensations I'd only imagined, I didn't spare a single thought for how my body looked—I just reveled in the things it was able to feel. Believe me, I know it's easier said than done, but the more you can focus on what your body can do and feel, the more it will take you out of worrying about how it looks.

My background also includes years of theater, both onstage and backstage. I've had to audition more times than I can count, and the best advice I ever received was not to make any excuses or disclaimers. So many performers would get onstage and say, "Sorry, I have a cold, my voice is scratchy," before launching into their song. Most of the time, they sounded great. And if they hadn't made an excuse, you'd never have known something was wrong. But once they said something like that, you'd be looking out for it. You'd be listening for the edge of a scratch in their voice. And you wouldn't be focusing on what an amazing performer they were.

My weak point was always dance. I'm hopelessly

uncoordinated and also slightly dyslexic, so memorizing choreography was a waking nightmare. But many of the auditions required song, dance, and monologue. So I had to muddle through.

Again, the advice I received was not to apologize, but just to sell the hell out of it. So I'd get up there and I'd plaster a huge smile on my face, make eye contact with the judges, and wait for my music cue. As I danced I'd know I was messing up the steps. Missing things entirely, failing to land jumps—just about any way a dance could go wrong, I'd find. But I'd keep that smile on my face the whole time, and I'd make smiling eye contact with the judges every time I faced forward, and I'd smile and bow when it was over.

I never landed a dance-heavy part (thank goodness), but I got cast in plenty of roles that spoke to my strengths. At one audition one of the directors even commented on my system, saying, "Pretty sure you missed every step in that dance, but you looked so happy doing it, I didn't care." And that's what it all comes down to: confidence. Or at least selling the image of confidence when you aren't quite feeling it yet.

A couple things happen when you act confident, even when you don't one hundred percent feel it—you convince your audience, and you begin to convince yourself.

Just like the constant negative self-talk takes its toll on us, because we believe it, the performance of confidence also begins to sink in, and we start to believe it. Studies have been done to show that looking in the mirror and giving yourself positive affirmations helps your self-esteem, even if you feel silly while you're doing it. The same is true for adjusting your posture to something more confident. They've shown that if you hold a super-hero pose—hands on your hips, chest out—for a couple minutes before going to speak onstage, you'll have more confidence and more stage presence.

The first step to addressing negative self-talk is to notice that it's happening. It's kind of like noticing yourself breathing or blinking (you're doing it now, aren't you?). Once you've noticed it, it's hard to stop. So now I bet you'll catch yourself the next time you have a negative thought about yourself. And that's great! Once you've noticed that it's happening, you can interrupt the thought.

The next step is to acknowledge that the feeling is real and valid, but not objective reality. Your fears are normal, but they won't necessarily come to pass, and the way you see yourself likely isn't the way others see you. Take as long as you need at this step to get in the habit of catching and interrupting these thoughts when they happen.

Then, when you're ready, start replacing the negative thoughts with positive ones. This is the trickiest part, but there's good news—even if you feel silly, or don't entirely believe the new positive statements, they're still effective.

What does any of this have to do with sex? Everything.

All too often we're afraid to undress in front of a partner because we don't like how we look. Or we're deciding what sex acts to do based on how flattering we think they'll be for us. But all of this is taking us out of our bodies and into our heads, and making it so we don't enjoy sex as much, if at all.

And you know what? I can just about guarantee that your partner hasn't noticed or doesn't care about that thing that's got you feeling self-conscious. We're always our harshest critics, and affection creates its own rose-colored glasses through which we view our partners. In fact, your partner might even love that thing that you hate about your body.

So here are some guidelines, should you care to follow them:

- Don't make any excuses or disclaimers. This starts with dating profiles and profile pictures. Whatever you're presenting, present it with confidence.
- Don't bring body negativity on your dates or into your bedroom.
- Find things to wear that make you feel sexy, and then just go with it. Once you've made the decision of what to wear, don't second-guess it.
- If you need reassurances that your partner likes the way you look, it's okay to ask for them—just couch them in positive terms, and no trick questions!
- Remember that if you're being critical about your body, or about other people's bodies (strangers, celebrities), you'll likely make your partner worry what you think of their body.
- Perform confidence, even when feeling it is a work in progress. Confidence rates as one of the sexiest traits, so just sell whatever you're doing with a big smile.

Start having the kind of sex you want right now. Don't wait for anything to change. I sit in my office hearing from clients who regret how long they waited to do the things they want; I never hear from people who regret trying something before they lost a few pounds. And if you're not there yet, that's okay, too. Everyone deserves love and hot sex, no matter where they're at with self-love and body confidence.

"FAILED" SEX

I don't believe sex can be a failure. And I don't believe in setting ourselves up with goals that can make us feel we've failed. This can be tricky, because some sex acts might seem like they're all or nothing. Like either you've done the thing, or you haven't.

I've been there, too. The first time I asked someone to fist me, I was determined to get them wrist-deep, and I probably would have felt like I failed if I didn't make it. Even though that act seems like a special case, with subsequent partners I've made it clear that even if they're trying to fist me, I want it to be about the whole experience, and I want them ready to pivot to another activity if that one isn't working for me.

Having a backup plan is one of the best ways to avoid feeling like you've failed. Having a plan B, C, and even D means that you can try several new things and keep moving on to something else if they don't work for you.

This can become especially important in long-term relationships, when it's easy to feel a lot of pressure on how your sex life is going. If you're not connecting in a sexual way very often, it can feel even scarier to try something and not have it go as planned. Having a broader definition of sex and intimacy also helps with this. Because then if nothing else, you haven't had failed sex, you've had successful intimacy.

Some people define sex in a way that sets them up for failure (or pressures a partner into faking responses). If you're basing your idea of sex on what movies have shown you, you might think that mind-blowing simultaneous orgasms are the only way that good sex can go.

But not everyone is always going to have an orgasm, simultaneous or otherwise. And feeling pressure to have one can make them even less likely. Not only that, but putting too much emphasis on orgasms can make people less willing to have sex when they think they might not be able to climax. And then they, and their partner, are missing out on all the other yummy intimacy that can occur.

Throughout our lifetimes, many of us will experience conditions that change the way our bodies respond sexually, from childbirth to aging to changes in physical and mental health to simply experiencing accidents or injuries. If we have rigid ideas about sex and consider everything else a failure, these changes can feel like even more of a loss.

Focusing on the wide range of ways we can feel pleasure and intimacy makes all kinds of encounters successful.

ANATOMY LESSON

In order to talk about our bodies, we need to know what's going on with our bodies! Part of what's lacking from most sex ed is any talk about pleasure. So if we know about anatomy at all, it's usually from the point of view of procreation, not what feels good.

University studies have shown that among people with vulvas, only roughly twenty-six percent have taken a close look. I'm talking "get cozy with a mirror" close. And while that number feels shockingly low to me, the state of sexual health in our culture seems to bear it out.

Information about sex, and sexual anatomy, is political. Information about bodies has come and gone from textbooks over the centuries, heavily influenced by the morality of the time. Some of this information has only resurfaced in the last few decades.

For people with vulvas, there's a lot going on that you can't see from the outside. The clitoral complex, and in fact the whole clitoral-urethral-vaginal complex, is an elaborate system that ties together to make a variety of forms of pleasure possible.

Even the words surrounding bodies can be misleading. Most books refer to labia majora and labia minora, but built right into the names is the assumption that the minora are smaller, which is often not the case. For this reason, educators usually say inner and outer lips.

Choices of language like that matter, because if the mainstream terms don't fit a person, that leaves them feeling damaged or wrong in some way, and those feelings have real-life consequences.

Even though bodies might look different from the outside, there are more similarities than you might realize. For one thing, there's the same amount of erectile tissue in the clitoral complex as there is in a penis. One is just far more visible outside the body.

It's well worth picking up a book that focuses on anatomy (see the resources section for suggestions), as this section is only an overview. Also, the science that we do have around the sexual function of our bodies is sorely lacking. It becomes especially complex when discussing the vulva, vagina, clitoris, and surrounding structures.

"The anatomical structures that might provoke vaginally activated orgasms rather than clitorally activated orgasms have not been completely and unequivocally described, probably representing a unique case of remaining major uncertainty regarding human gross anatomy . . . Whether the Gräfenberg spot is a discrete entity, a complex structure, or a gynaecological myth created for journalistic purposes, or with the aim of supporting surgical aesthetic manipulations of the female genitals, remains unclear. [Furthermore] the existence of the vaginally activated orgasm, based on the opinion or experiences of a number of women, has often been rejected, largely for political rather than scientific reasons."[4]

Although the details are still debated, what is sure is that many people experience great pleasure and orgasm from having the area of their vaginal wall commonly called the G-spot stimulated. We are now seeing that this area is more accurately described as the clitourethrovaginal (CUV) complex.

For people with penises, whether or not they've been circumcised can play a role in how sensitive they are and the ways they like to be touched. The frenulum is often very sensitive—as to whether this is a good thing or a bad thing, you'll have to ask the person it's attached to.

The same is true for the clitoral glans, the part of the clit that you can see outside the body. For some people it's too sensitive for direct stimulation. For others, a great deal of intense stimulation is necessary for pleasure.

We think we know where most of the pleasure centers

---

4   Jannini, E. A., Buisson, O., Rubio-Casillas, A., "Beyond the G Spot: Clitourethrovaginal Complex Anatomy in Female Orgasm," *Nature Reviews Urology* 11,, no. 9 (2014): 531–538; published online 12 August 2014. doi:10.1038/nrurol.2014.193.

of the genitals are, but they're far more varied and complex than you might realize. And everyone is different. For some people, their labia are more sensitive or more receptive to pleasurable touch than their clitoris.

For some people, the scrotum is an area of untapped enjoyment, and for others this area might be too sensitive or ticklish.

While anal play or anal sex might be considered taboo by some, it's also an area of the body with a lot of sensitive nerve endings, and an area that can receive a great deal of pleasure. Simply exploring around the outside of the anus can be an intensely pleasurable feeling, and you can stop there if penetration doesn't sound appealing.

If you do want to try anal penetration, know that this area is so sensitive, every movement can be felt acutely, and you don't need much girth to make an impact. Exploring with a single finger or with a toy made for anal play is a great way to get started. Curved toys are pleasurable for many people, as they help stimulate either the prostate or the G-spot. (Yes, you can stimulate the CUV region from the anal cavity!)

Anal penetration generally goes past the first two sphincters, the one you can see when you look at the body, and a second internal sphincter that you can't consciously control. At the other end of the rectum is a third sphincter, leading to the colon, and it's best not to explore that far when you're playing. Not only would that enhance the likelihood of causing harm, but at that point there aren't very sensitive receptors for pleasure, so there isn't anything to be gained.

Pleasure anatomy isn't just about the genitals. Our whole bodies from tip to toe can experience exquisite pleasure, and it's your (fun!) job to find all the places on your body, and on partners' bodies, that are the most enjoyable.

For every body part I can list, there will be some people who love having it touched or played with and other people it leaves cold. There's no way around asking and experimenting. But it helps to know the general layout so you know what things are on the menu to try.

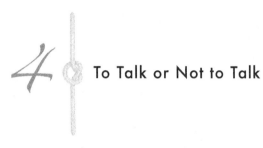

4   To Talk or Not to Talk

WHEN TO TALK

MAKING TIME TO TALK

THIS MIGHT SOUND SILLY, BUT WE DON'T ALWAYS make time to talk to the people who are the most important to us. Maybe you chat about your day, what's going on at the office, or the movie you just saw, but when did you last talk about your feelings?

Or maybe you and your sweetie(s) don't get to see each other that often, and you feel reluctant to "ruin" date night by having hard conversations. You just want to enjoy your time together and not risk derailing the evening.

Either way, sometimes the most important things are the hardest to bring up.

Whether you're simply giving your partner a heads-up that there's something you'd like to talk about and asking if it's a good time, or actually scheduling time to talk, it's important to differentiate "talks" from simply chatting about your day.

You need to be in a different head space to really share—and hear—heavier stuff about how you or a partner are feeling. That's why it can be helpful to have a scheduled time on the calendar to talk about how things are going. Depending what your organizational style is, you can even make an agenda for these talks.

Whether you set these talks for once a week or once a month, it can be helpful to know that you've got a time coming when you can raise any concerns you've been having, set your shared schedule for the coming week or month, and make sure you're on the same page about the relationship.

If you're a note-taking type, like I am, you might even keep a running list for yourself of things you want to talk about at the next meeting. Putting something on the list and knowing you'll get a chance to sort through whatever it is can help take it off your mind in the meantime.

When you have your first scheduled relationship talk, set some ground rules about how you'd like it to go. Are you agreeing on an agenda together? Are you each getting equal time? Are you tackling one big topic, then each adding your own smaller items that have come up since the last meeting? Knowing how the talk will go can be as important as the talks themselves.

Another thing to consider is location. Some people will be most comfortable doing this at home, and for other people having these talks in public is easier. Sometimes being out in the world is a good backdrop to keep things on an even keel, if you're afraid the talk might get tense or emotional.

The bottom line is figuring out what it takes logistically to make it most likely that you and your sweetie(s) will get what you need from these conversations.

At a minimum, give your partner a heads-up when you want to have a difficult conversation, and check in about whether it's a good time. Sure, sometimes things come up in the moment that have to be addressed, but if the issue isn't immediate, you'll get the best results if you have the conversation when everyone is in the right head space for it. It's also another way to establish a consent culture within your relationship, by letting people opt in to serious talks rather than being surprised by them.

With clients, I often call these State of the Relationship talks. Just like oil changes, software updates, and putting air in the tires, everything requires ongoing maintenance, and relationships are no exception. Once you've decided to have these regular talks, here are some things you might want to cover:

▸ Needs and definitions around sex.
▸ Household logistics, chores, etc.
▸ Vacation planning.
▸ Big personal topics that affect everyone—job changes, moves, etc.
▸ Your schedule for the coming week or month, depending how often you have these talks.
▸ Scheduling date nights.

Sometimes just knowing that you have a built-in space coming up to raise issues can make things feel less urgent. Often it's not knowing when or how to bring something up that causes the most stress. When you have these talks already on the schedule, you'll also have a built-in time for bringing up new kinds of sex you'd like to try, or a fantasy you'd like to tell your partner about.

Most people think that figuring out how to start the conversation is the hardest part, so if you've got time to talk built in already, you've already done the hardest part and you can focus on the information you want to share, rather than worrying about how to bring it up.

PUTTING IT IN WRITING

Have you ever thought something was perfectly clear, only to realize that someone else thought something completely different? It's happened to all of us at one time or another. One way to help avoid this is to keep explicit agreements written down. This could mean a journal that's kept somewhere that all involved parties have access to, or it could be a shared Google document—whatever works best for you and the people involved. Regardless of the format, having things written down can be helpful in a few ways.

The act of writing things down forces you to make sure that the same understanding has been reached. When you discuss what's getting written down, you can find out if you're on the same page—literally. And this clarity goes a long way toward avoiding miscommunications. Having agreements written down also helps make sure that the vagaries of memory won't cause trouble later on.

Perhaps you've heard the saying that there are three versions of every story: my version, your version, and the truth. This isn't about people lying or being intentionally manipulative. It's simply how memory works sometimes. That's why eyewitness accounts of crimes are notoriously unreliable. So having agreements in writing, that you can refer to, removes some of the memory guesswork.

So what kinds of topics or agreements lend themselves to a written record? Let's examine a few.

Making plans

Do you have an agreed-upon date night? Did you get tickets to a concert? Have a shared calendar or schedule, whether it's paper on the wall or something shared online. Be clear about what's been agreed to so feelings don't get hurt.

This goes for holidays, birthdays, and anniversaries, too. Pop culture would lead you to believe you're supposed to be a mind reader around these events—but that's a great way to wind up with frustration and hurt feelings all around. If you're expecting to spend a particular day with a partner, be sure you've talked about it.

Safer-sex agreements

You want to make sure your safer-sex agreements are crystal clear. Sometimes it can help to get them down on paper to make sure everyone's understandings are exactly the same. These agreements can include how often STI testing will occur, what kind of barriers will be used during sexual activity, and what kind of communication and disclosure will happen between partners.

Household duties

If you live with someone, it can be helpful to have clarity about who has agreed to do what. Avoid arguments on trash day by having all agreements in writing and easily accessible.

These are just a few examples. What's important to you might look completely different. But keep in mind that these agreements are likely to change over time and should be revisited on a regular basis. Writing them down is for the sake of clarity, not so that they're set in stone and can never be changed.

SCHEDULING

For people with busy lives, scheduling can be not only stressful, but a sore point in relationships. Not only scheduling dates, but scheduling time for sex. People may roll their eyes at that and think that eliminating the spontaneity takes the fun out of sex, but is that really worse than not having sex at all?

Here's where we can take a lesson from kinksters or swingers—communities where planning parties and play is the norm. When you have something on the calendar in advance, you have a chance to look forward to it, to plan, and discuss, and maybe choose outfits or toys. Rather than ruining the fun, it builds anticipation.

It can also take some of the pressure off if you simply plan for connective or intimate time. There doesn't have to be any particular kind of sex, or any sex at all. But when the people involved have busy lives, you may be surprised how much time can go by without spending quality time together before you start to notice something amiss.

Scheduling can work a lot of different ways. You can take a cue from the polyamory community and use Google Calendar, or if you live with the person you're scheduling with, maybe you have a whiteboard calendar on the fridge. Whatever technology works for you, try to make sure you've got scheduled dates.

To help make this fun rather than a chore, try keeping a running list of things you'd like to do on your dates together. This can include restaurants to try, concerts or movies to see, or sex stores to explore together. Whenever you see an interesting Facebook event pop up, or something listed in the newspaper grabs your attention, you can add it to this running list you share. Then when you sit down to do your scheduling or have your State of the Relationship talk, you'll already have some ideas of what to do together, and ideally the dates will be things you're looking forward to.

Frequency of dates or sex is a common sore point in relationships. Just like everything else, it's important to talk to your partner or partners about your expectations in these areas, to help prevent frustration or hurt feelings. In a future chapter, we'll discuss mismatched levels of desire, but for now we're talking simple logistics.

If you and your partner would like to be having more sex, but jobs, kids, and life are getting in the way, how can you arrange your schedule to make sure there's time for intimacy? Sometimes economics doesn't allow for working shorter hours or hiring a babysitter. But making time for intimacy should make its way onto the list of priorities when you're scheduling and budgeting.

To make this easier, it helps if you feel like you're in this together. It's not one person trying to get something from the other person, it's the two of you trying to work this out together. And keep in mind that not every date needs to be a whole day or a whole evening. You can get creative and find ways to make shorter time meaningful, too.

Whether it's fitting lunch or coffee into a workday or taking some ideas from the long-distance relationships section to use Skype or texting as a way to maintain intimacy, feel free to get creative about how you stay connected to your partner.

WHEN NOT TO TALK

WHEN TO PROCESS WITH A FRIEND, NOT A PARTNER

Often, our partners become our main go-to people when we want to process our feelings, from what happened at work that day to struggles with our friends to issues with housing. But what about when the issues or feelings you're having are *about* your partner? Or, in the case of an open relationship, about one of your other partners?

Sometimes it's more appropriate to reach out to a friend.

Even when you're reaching out to a friend rather than a partner, it's helpful to follow some of the same procedures we've talked about. Ask your friend if they've got the time and bandwidth to process with you. And make sure you let them know if you just want an ear, a shoulder to cry on, or if you want help brainstorming solutions.

Before talking to a friend, think about what you need to share to get help, and what should stay private. For these decisions it can be best to have explicit conversations with your partner about what can be shared and what stays between the two of you. For example, sometimes details of sex acts or fantasies might be too intimate to share. But keep in mind that you can always talk about your own experience, and if someone is trying to keep you quiet, or keep you from talking to your friends, that can be a big red flag.

Also keep in mind that if you find yourself regularly going to friends to talk about your partner, that might indicate a problem, too. If you're frequently complaining *about* someone, rather than talking *to* them, that's not a great sign.

When sharing with friends, remember to share the positive, as well as the challenging, things about your relationship. Most people are prone to complain more than to share happy moments. That doesn't mean the happy moments aren't there, it just doesn't always occur to us to tell people about them. Maybe we don't want to sound like we're gloating, or it's just that misery loves company. But make sure you're not turning your friends against your partner by only sharing the negative.

If you bring up a problem to a friend—whether they give you advice or not—it might be a good idea to circle back and let them know how that issue ended up being resolved, so they know it isn't still pending.

Sharing the good things, and keeping your friends informed of the balance of your relationship, will also help them give better advice, or at least be a more neutral listener, when you do need to lean on them. If they only ever hear the negative, they might not understand why you're in the relationship, or be tempted to suggest you end things.

WHEN TO GET OUTSIDE HELP

Sometimes we need to seek professional help, and that's

okay. There are some issues that can't be solved with all the communication skills in the world. Whether that means individual or couples' therapy or coaching, there are a wide variety of sex-positive professionals to choose from.

How do you know when it's time to get professional support? Any time you've tried the tools at your disposal and you're still feeling stuck, it's worth looking into.

Couples counseling

When things have stagnated for a while and you can't seem to get conversations started, or when you aren't talking to each other at all, professional help may get your communication jump-started.

Not only do therapists, counselors, and coaches have a variety of tools at their disposal, but going to see someone means making time in your schedule for the talks and being in the neutral space of their office. Sometimes just those two factors make it both worth going and incredibly helpful.

Going to see someone as a couple can be like having your State of the Relationship talk with a neutral third party, or with a moderator/mediator. Having someone else in the room who can help set the container of what's going to be covered, and making sure conversations stay on topic, can be a huge help. They can make sure that each person has time to talk and time to address their feelings, and they can help ensure that everyone is hearing each other and understanding what's being said.

Sometimes the reframing of an issue that a trained third party can offer makes all the difference if you've been coming at the issue from the same angle for months or years. As can simply making the commitment to see someone and show that you're both invested in working things out.

When there's been a breach of trust or relationship agreements, and emotions are running high, having a neutral third party keep the conversation going and on track can be a valuable resource.

Individual counseling

If you've never been to therapy, give it a try. Although the stigma is starting to fade, many people still avoid this kind of help for fear it means they're "crazy." It doesn't mean that at all. Therapists and counselors are simply experts in a certain field, and you should reach out to them the same way you'd get professional help in any other field, like having someone manage your finances or file your taxes.

Having an outside perspective, even if you're not dealing with any particular diagnosis, can be incredibly valuable. And if there are not mental health issues at hand, other helping professionals like coaches can be a great option.

Wondering how to know if you should get help? Here are a few examples of why you might want to seek a counselor or therapist, but any time you're struggling is a good time to get support.

▸ If you're feeling consistently overwhelmed, or you feel like your responses to situations are out of proportion to what happened.
▸ When you feel like you're having a hard time keeping up with your responsibilities.
▸ When you're recovering from trauma.
▸ Substance use/self-medicating.
▸ You've experienced a big loss.

▸ You're not enjoying things you used to enjoy.
▸ Friends/partners/family express worry about you.

Relationships are made up of people, and each person must address their own issues and take care of themselves if they want the relationship to be healthy. Sometimes taking a pause to work on individual issues is the best thing that can happen to a relationship.

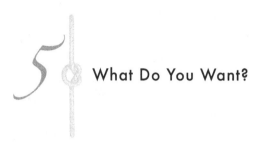

What Do You Want?

GET IN TOUCH WITH YOURSELF

IF YOU'RE GOING TO COMMUNICATE WHAT YOU do and don't want to a partner, you have to know what you do and don't want. And that isn't as easy as it sounds, because so much of our programming is about pleasing other people and fitting in that we've often forgotten how to listen to our bodies. From being told to finish all the food on our plates to being forced to receive kisses or pinches on the cheek from that aunt or uncle who creeped us out, we often spend our formative years being forced to ignore the things our body is telling us, and then at some magical point (maybe our eighteenth birthday?), bodily autonomy is apparently bestowed upon us. Well, by then we've learned some bad habits.

Maybe this sounds silly, but we need to relearn what our yeses and noes feel like. You can start doing that work right now, just by listening to your body.

When I'm teaching classes on consent and boundaries,

I encourage people to get up out of their seats and move around to try a few things. One of my favorite exercises is one where you can find the outline of your personal bubble. It's going to be different for different people and in different situations. For example, it might be a much smaller bubble with intimate partners and close friends and a much bigger bubble with complete strangers.

In classes I encourage people to divide into two groups. The As get to be the first ones calling the shots. The Bs stand across the room from them and begin approaching slowly. As they approach, the As need to decide how close they want to let the other person get before asking them to stop. Most As stop the Bs anywhere from one to three feet away from them.

The point of the exercise is to feel what it's like in your body as someone is getting close. At what point does it start to feel awkward or uncomfortable? At what point do you start to feel the urge to take a step back? And where do you feel that discomfort? Is it a tightness in your chest, butterflies in your stomach, or something else? When you start learning to identify that feeling, you can look out for it all the time, and then you can do a better job of setting the best boundaries for you.

While you can certainly recruit people to do this exercise with you, you can also do it on your own in everyday life. Next time you're standing in line at the grocery store or at the bank, think about how closely you're standing to the next person in line. Why did you choose that distance? What if you go to a bar and need to squeeze between two people to order a drink? How much space does there need to be for you to go for it and wedge yourself in, and when would you just stand back and wait?

Your answers to all of these questions will be influenced by a number of factors, and gender is probably a big one. How close we're willing to be to other people is often influenced by whether or not we think they're a threat. So you can think about that as well while you're doing your personal sociological experiments in your daily life.

You can pay attention to your yeses and noes in other parts of your life, too. What about when someone offers you something to eat or drink? Aside from accepting out of politeness, what happens when you're being offered something that you love versus something you're not crazy about?

The point is to develop a really solid understanding of how our bodies respond so we can check in with ourselves as we're doing the following exercises and talking to partners about sex. Because we only want to say yes to things we're genuinely excited about, things that we are as into as being offered our favorite dessert. If you're not excited about the thing you're being offered, there's always something else to try instead.

EXPLORING YOUR OPTIONS

One common question that comes up in sex-ed classes and with sex coaching clients is how to ask for what you want when you don't know what you want. For a variety of reasons, people don't always know what their options are. Many people come of age absent any useful information about sex and have only locker-room whispers to guide them. In fact, it's not uncommon for someone to get to midlife, or older, and realize they aren't really enjoying their sex life. It's easy for that to be pushed aside in favor of career, family, or any other ways we've prioritized our time.

Maybe there's a big life change that encourages people to start prioritizing sex and sexuality. Maybe it's after a breakup that people start wondering what else is out there. Or they've just started a new relationship that's more sexually open than they're used to, and now that exploring is possible, they need help knowing where to start.

Whether you're in a long-term relationship and you want to change things up a little or you're young or new to dating and just want to get off on the right foot, it's never too early—or too late—to prioritize your sexual expression and enjoyment. And you've come to the right place. There are many tools at your disposal to help you figure out what kinds of sex, sexuality, and intimacy you might enjoy.

Through the following exercises, you'll start to discover what you might like to learn about and explore, and what's a hard limit for you.

FUTURE PERFECT

In coaching, one of the tools we're trained to use with clients is the "future perfect" exercise. You think about where you'd like to be in five or ten years and you do a writing exercise where you explore exactly what this looks like. For some people, it's very general. But coaches are trained to help people dig down into specifics. Imagine a day in that perfect life. What's the first thing you hear when you wake up? What do you have for breakfast? In exacting detail, move through your whole day. In this way details about your home, your family, your job, and more will come to light. It can help our brains figure out the bigger-picture stuff when we're focusing on the details.

You can do this exercise for your sex life, too. Think

about what your ideal sex life would be. If you want, you can do the more general version. Think about how often you'd like to be having sex, what sex acts you'd like to engage in, and how you'd like to feel. But it's most valuable if you really dig into details. Imagine a whole scenario from beginning to end. Consider as many details as you can:

> ▸ What are you wearing?
> ▸ Who are you with?
> ▸ Where are you?
> ▸ Is there a bed? What is it like?
> ▸ Describe your setting.
> ▸ What do you smell?
> ▸ What do you hear?
> ▸ What kind of lighting is there?
> ▸ How do you feel in your body?
> ▸ In detail, what do you do? How does each thing make you feel?

You can get as detailed and creative as you'd like. It doesn't matter if some (or all) of it seems unrealistic. We'll address that later. For now, you're in pure fantasy mode. We just want to get as many of your desires as possible out of your subconscious and onto the paper. This is the more difficult part. Once you know what you want, you can make a plan to get there.

Don't let fears about your writing get in your way. The finished product doesn't have to read like erotica. If it helps you to get words on the page, you can simply use a list format, or do this exercise like a mind map.

You never need to show anyone what you've written,

so give yourself permission to write badly. And I'll let you in on a secret—that's the same tactic professional authors use. First drafts are supposed to be terrible—it's just about getting the thoughts and ideas on the page. And that's what you're doing here. You're using the process of writing to mine your subconscious for ideas about what you'd like to experience. That's where the value is. It doesn't matter if what you write makes sense. Spelling, grammar, narrative—not the point. As long as you understand what you're getting at, that's all that matters.

WHAT ARE YOUR HIGHLIGHTS?

You can have a fulfilling sex life and still have room for exploration and even improvement. There's always something new to try. And calling on your past positive experiences can be one of the best ways to figure out what to do going forward. Another coaching tool I've adapted for sex is that of figuring out what's working so you can do more of that.

If you know that when you're well rested and well fed you do your best work, you'll strive to be well rested and well fed on a regular basis. Sure, it can be tricky with our busy lives and busy schedules to always take the best care of ourselves, but if you know that's optimal for you, it's a goal you work toward.

In that example, you know what works well for you and try to do more of that.

So in your sex life, what's already working that you'd like more of? This exercise doesn't have to be limited to your current sex life or partners. For this, you can think about all the sexual experiences you've ever had. What felt the best? What was the most satisfying? The most fulfilling? Like our last exercise, it helps to think in as much detail as possible.

When you think of your best sexual encounters, what were the factors? What stood out as amazing? Was it the setting? The person or people you were with? The physical acts you were engaging in? How you felt, emotionally or physically?

See if you can notice the patterns among your favorite encounters. Were they all when you were on vacation? Or when you had lots of time to explore and indulge? Maybe they were all public bathroom quickies. Whatever it is for you, notice the patterns so you can start to replicate them.

Here are some questions you can ask yourself to get you started:

▸ If you have orgasms, what was the best/strongest orgasm you remember having? What was going on when it happened?
▸ When do you remember feeling the most safe?
▸ When do you remember feeling the most comfortable?
▸ When do you remember feeling the most turned on?
▸ When was the last time you felt butterflies in your stomach, or were so excited to try something you could hardly wait?
▸ What experience(s) have you had that you couldn't wait to tell a friend about?
▸ What have you done with a partner or partners that you looked back on fondly with them?
▸ When did you feel like something was naughty/exciting/taboo?

> ▸ What was the longest you ever spent having sex/
> intimacy?
> ▸ What was your quickest sexual encounter?
> ▸ Have you had an encounter after being separated
> from a partner for a while? What was that like?

These questions are simply to help you start thinking about the sex you've had, to help you remember high points. Keep in mind that a whole encounter doesn't have to be amazing for one feature of it to be worth repeating, so keep an open mind as you sort through your memories.

SENSATIONS EXERCISE

Whether because you don't have a lot of existing experiences to pull from, or they simply haven't been optimal, sometimes the best way to start exploring is simply to close your eyes and fantasize. Think about what sensations you want to experience and how you want to feel. Do you like the idea of soft and sensual, or rough and hard? Once you have an idea of how you want to feel, it can be easier to think of the ways you might be able to achieve those feelings.

Here's an incomplete list of feelings and sensations for you to ponder. As you read through the list, there are a few things you can do. First, it can be helpful to close your eyes and think about each one in turn. Give yourself enough time with each word to really feel it and think about your physical or emotional responses. As you start to figure out which ones appeal to you the most, you can star them in the list (maybe with pencil) or make your own separate list of what's most appealing to you right now. Because in another day, week, month, or year, your list might be completely different.

- Tender
- Sensitive
- Tight
- Restricted
- Held
- Soft
- Cool
- Warm
- Sharp
- Intense
- Bitten
- Penetrated
- Hot
- Plush
- Disheveled
- Eager
- Shameless
- Breathless
- Squirmy
- Tingly
- Electric
- Dark

- Bright
- Teased
- Massaged
- Loud
- Silky
- Quiet
- Aching
- Sweaty
- Calm
- Captured
- Supported
- Afterglow
- Safe
- Exhilarated
- Secure
- Aroused
- Lingering
- Naughty
- Curious
- Ticklish
- Shy
- Acute

Add your own words as you think of them either during the exercise or throughout your day. You can also come back to the list after you've had a sexual experience and try to add any feelings or sensations you just experienced so that you'll remember what's possible. Then you can also decide which of those sensations you'd like more of in the future, and which ones you'd like to modify.

When you've got a list of three to five things you'd like to experience, then you can do the creative work of building a scene around them. For each sensation you'd like to experience, think of the ways you can get there.

If the word *soft* appeals to you, that could mean lying on soft sheets while you play, or having soft fabrics or furs gliding along your skin. It could mean soft touches from a partner, or even music playing softly in the background. As you think of ways to bring these sensations to life, you may also find ways to more closely pinpoint what you're looking for.

Whatever words you choose, play with building a scene around them. I'm not going to do the math, but I think you'd be busy for the rest of your life if you tried every possible combination of three to five of these sensations.

YES/NO/MAYBE

One of the most straightforward ways to start thinking about what you might like to try is with a yes/no/maybe list. Perhaps you've heard of them before. Sometimes they're called sexual inventory checklists. They're especially common in the kink scene, but there are versions for all kinds of sexual and connective activities.

Just like going to a restaurant or bar and looking through the menu, you can read about each option and decide whether it sounds good to you right now. And like perusing a dessert menu after a filling meal, you can also decide there are things you want to come back and try another time.

These lists provide a starting point where you can

think about all the ways people can express sexuality or kink, alone or with a partner or partners, and decide what you'd like to try. The lists aren't a substitute for talking with your partner, but they are a fantastic tool for brainstorming and negotiating. And when you come upon items you've never heard of or never considered, it gives you a starting point for researching some of your options.

When you're using these lists with a partner, you can each fill out your list and then compare notes. The mutual yeses are an easy place to start, but it's valuable to talk about the maybe and no answers, too. It's not about trying to change someone's mind. But it can be valuable to know why someone feels the way they do about various activities.

For one thing, it's a great time to see if you both have the same definitions for the terms. Even for mutual yeses, you should talk about what you mean, to make sure everyone is on the same page.

When it comes to items on the no list, those can be valuable conversations, too. Maybe someone has put an item in the no list because of a bad experience they had. For example, I often hear people say they aren't interested in anal play or anal sex because of one bad experience. When you get more information about that, it's often a youthful exploration that wasn't done with much preparation, let alone lube. If that's what they're thinking of when you bring up anal play, of course it won't sound appealing. But a gentle exploration with a mouth or well-lubed finger, just focusing on external stimulation, might be another story altogether.

If you want, you can just read through the lists below to get an idea of what's possible—things you might want to research or talk about. Or you can use this as a worksheet and circle or star your yeses (maybe in pencil, because things do change). Or write your own yes, no, and maybe columns in a notebook and add these items to the appropriate columns.

Pay attention to your reactions as you're going through the lists. Do some ideas turn you on? Do others scare you? Are there things you feel like you "should" want for a partner, but you're not into them? All of these feelings are valuable to know about and will help you when you're talking to partners.

Keep in mind, some of these things might sound hot to you—and you still might not want to do them. And that's totally fine. Lots of people have fantasies that are just that, fantasies. We all have some turn-ons, some things we like to think about, that we don't necessarily ever want to do in real life. Some of these things become topics we want to fantasize about with a partner, maybe work them into dirty talk, or erotica or porn selection, and some of them just stay fantasies for ourselves.

You can also use these lists to negotiate for each encounter. It can be helpful to know what kinds of play you'll want to do on each date, as these lists are almost sure to change from day to day and week to week. The things we're in the mood for, and the things our bodies are up for, can vary a lot. So it's never safe to assume that just because someone liked a certain activity last time you saw them, they'll be up for the same thing this time.

Ready to get started? This isn't an exhaustive list, but it's a good starting point for deciding what to explore.

- Kissing
- Necking
- Public displays of affection
- Sexual touch in public or semipublic
- Being seen naked by a partner/seeing a partner naked
- Touching yourself in front of a partner
- Watching your partner touch themselves
- Tickling/being tickled
- Giving or receiving massage
- Dirty talk
- Sharing fantasies
- Frottage
- Hand sex, external
- Hand sex, penetrative
- Hand sex, anal
- Ejaculation on your body/on your partner's body
- Ejaculation in your body/in your partner's body

- Analingus/rimming/oral-anal contact
- Using sex toys alone
- Using sex toys with a partner
- Performing oral sex
- Receiving oral sex
- Penetrative vaginal intercourse, giving or receiving
- Penetrative anal intercourse, giving or receiving
- Playing with food
- Cross-dressing
- Biting/being bitten
- Scratching
- Leaving marks/bruises
- Bondage
- Blindfolds
- Strap-on play
- Pegging
- Playing with ice cubes
- Face slapping
- Role-playing
- Phone sex
- Sexting
- Cybersex
- Video sex

- Watching porn alone or with a partner
- Reading erotica alone or with a partner
- Spanking
- Paddles
- Floggers
- Canes
- Whips
- Riding crops
- Clothespins
- Playing with power, domination, and submission
- Nipple play or nipple clamps
- Orgasm control, tease and denial, asking for permission to orgasm
- Threesomes
- Group sex
- Sex parties
- BDSM parties
- Gags
- Hair pulling
- Playing with hot wax
- Electrical play
- Water sports/urine play
- Wearing a collar
- Taking photos
- Taking videos
- Sex or play outdoors
- Exhibitionism
- Voyeurism

Remember, having a mutual yes isn't the end of negotiation, it's the beginning. Does spanking mean a gentle tap or a hard swat? If you're having penetrative sex, are you using barriers? If you're having hand sex, are you using gloves?

You also need to discuss when and where the various activities are happening, and be explicit about whether they're always a yes, even without a check-in, or if you'd like to be asked first. For example, maybe it's always okay for your partner to kiss you without asking, but you want a heads-up before doing butt stuff.

Use this as a starting point, but don't forget to drill

into details. And be mindful of when and where you have these conversations. It can be helpful to have them well in advance of when sex or play might happen, and maybe to have them in a public place, too, so there's no pressure to try anything right away.

PULLING FANTASIES OUT OF MEDIA EXERCISE

As you're exploring your sexual fantasies and the things you might want to try, you may be surprised by how many fantasies are already lurking in your subconscious. We've all had things catch our eye during our lives, even if we didn't interpret them as sexual at the time.

Think about the images from magazines that you cut out and pinned to your wall in your teen years. For me, it was fashion spreads that invoked BDSM imagery. Or the page in a book that you dog-eared to read again and again, or to show to friends for the naughty thrill. Or the scene in a movie that you rewound to watch again and again. I remember being fascinated by things that I didn't completely understand, or being drawn to things that I might not have understood as sexual but that caught my attention all the same. Whether these items are overtly sexual for you, or simply scenes or images that invoke feelings you'd like to explore—all of those things are clues to what gets your juices flowing.

Many times we dismiss these things as unrealistic, unattainable, logistically impossible, or simply unsafe. And often, that's true. But these turn-ons can still become a great starting point for exploration. With a little thinking and creativity, you can find the essential features of a scenario that make it hot for you and work those elements into your real life.

When I'm teaching classes about finding your fantasy, I make myself vulnerable first, by sharing my own turn-ons, and then take volunteers from the audience. So here's how this exercise works for me:

When I was young, *Labyrinth* was one of my favorite movies. I watched it so many times I nearly wore out the VHS tape. And while David Bowie isn't going to whisk me away to a fantasy kingdom, I can still unlock a lot of clues to my sexuality thanks to him.

In case you're not familiar with the story, it goes something like this: Teenager Sarah is stuck babysitting her infant brother, Toby, and makes a wish to the goblin king that her brother will be taken away. But as soon as the goblins come, Sarah realizes her mistake and asks to have her brother back. This is when David Bowie, playing the goblin king, appears and where my own preteen fantasies began.

Bowie's character sets up a quest for Sarah, where she must find her way to his castle at the center of a labyrinth to retrieve her brother. This movie features power dynamics that are far from subtle. Each scene between Sarah and the goblin king is bristling with (unintentional?) tensions, and although I didn't have words for any of it at the time, I was clearly picking up on something. Bowie even carries a riding crop in at least one scene.

Sure, the details of a fantasy film might be challenging to replicate, but playing with power dynamics is easy. You don't need any toys or tools, just a little confidence, imagination, and a willingness to suspend disbelief.

Want to do some actual *Labyrinth* role play? Knock yourself out.

Just want to try giving or receiving orders? Simple to do!

The first step might simply be one person calling the shots. Or physically looming over the other person. Just putting one person on their knees sets up an immediate power imbalance that can be hot to explore. Add a little "do as I say" (with or without an attempt at Bowie's accent) and you've got my knees quaking.

What gets you going like that?

When I presented this class at a kink conference, my first volunteer decided to stick with the *Labyrinth* theme and brought up the scene where Sarah falls down a hole full of "helping hands." These hands grab at her and say they can guide her either up or down the passage. Does this scene get your attention, too? Think about the elements going on there.

The hands are anonymous.

There's pain, or at least discomfort.

There are multiple hands.

Sarah is out of control of the situation.

So, yes. The actual scene is difficult to replicate. But here's where we get creative. Think about how you could get the elements that are essential to this scene's hotness into your real life.

If you go to play parties, here's one way that could go:

You're tied down to a massage table (loss of control). You're blindfolded, making the people who touch you anonymous. Multiple people put their hands on your body. Some of them pinch or grab you.

Now that's a fairly literal interpretation, but that's because it's important to see that even seemingly outlandish fantasies might not be that hard to replicate.

What if you wanted to replicate it at home with only one partner? How about this:

You're blindfolded to help with the fantasy of anonymity. You could add bondage if you want to feel more vulnerable. Then, your partner touches you all over your body, pausing between touches so you don't know where you'll feel a hand next. Maybe your partner swaps out different kinds of gloves—latex, leather, fur—to provide various sensations. Maybe they use a few household objects to keep you off balance.

Depending on what pieces are essential to your turn-on, it's often a lot easier than you might think to work those elements into your sex life. I've interviewed dozens and dozens of people about their kinks and fetishes, asking them why they do the things they do. Regardless of the fetish, just about everyone had power, vulnerability, and trust on the list somewhere. And you don't need any special surroundings or equipment to play with those elements yourself.

Want to try the exercise on your own? Think about what caught your eye or turned you on at any time in your life. It could be from your childhood, like my example, or it could be a movie you saw last week. Write down what it is in the center of a piece of paper and draw a circle around it. Just a couple words so you know what you're talking about is fine. Then surround that circle with the elements of the scene or media that you find alluring. You can just jumble them all around the center circle or you can put the most essential elements closest to the middle and the bonus elements further out. Brainstorm for as long as it takes to figure out everything about it that turns you on or gets your attention.

Once you're satisfied with your list, start focusing on the elements independently of the original context. For example, if one of the elements is that a character is vulnerable, think about ways to create vulnerability in your own play. Here are a few ideas:

- ▸ Bondage
- ▸ Blindfolds
- ▸ Sensory deprivation (noise-canceling headphones, etc.)
- ▸ Being in unfamiliar surroundings. (This can be achieved at home by being blindfolded in one room and then led around so you don't know where you are anymore.)
- ▸ Verbally doing something scary, like sharing a fear or a secret.
- ▸ Letting someone take care of you in a personal or intimate way. (Being bathed, etc.)
- ▸ Relying on someone for something essential. (Being fed, etc.)

And these are just the ideas you can implement at home, with things you already have. When you start involving more people, or specialty locations, or props and toys, I'm sure you can think of many more.

PORN AND EROTICA

The idea of watching porn can be intimidating. You might not have any idea where to start, or if you've googled a few things, the top results might have been overwhelming or not to your taste. And it's true, porn isn't for everyone. But you might be surprised by what's actually available, and there could be something that's right up your alley. The resources section of this book lists several porn sites and producers you can start with. As much as possible, they've been screened for porn that's ethically produced— meaning the performers are paid well and treated well. Some people object to porn because they think it's exploitative, but that isn't always the case. You can even follow the results from the feminist porn awards if you want to keep up-to-date with new porn that's coming out.

If you want to go the slightly more old-fashioned way (or you're concerned about your internet browsing history) you can still get plenty of good porn on DVD. In fact, many sex-positive, all-gender-friendly sex toy stores have porn sections that you can browse. And the employees can likely point you in the right direction if you give them some idea of what you might be interested in.

Once you've decided what to start with, you'll have to decide if you want to watch alone or with a partner. Both options have their benefits—and you might decide to do both. If you're watching alone, sometimes that's a way to avoid self-consciousness. You can get an idea if you're into something before you choose to share it. When watching with a partner, the experience can be a turn-on if you're both into what you're watching. And watching together can also be a bonding experience, if doing so feels a little naughty or taboo.

Whether alone or together, pay attention to what you find arousing. What elements of the scenes do you like? Are there particular sex acts or positions you'd like to try? Does seeing one performer in a vulnerable, or powerful, stance appeal to you?

The caveat with porn is that it is fantasy entertainment.

Don't use porn as sex ed. You usually won't see the performers negotiating with each other, you won't always see them using lube, and you'll rarely see any kind of warm-up. The point of this exercise is not to duplicate what you see on the screen, but to see what catches your eye and then further research whatever that might be.

Maybe you see strap-on play or pegging in a porn scene and that gets your juices flowing. Great! Now, ignore how easily that toy likely slid inside the other performer, ignore the size of the toy, and ignore how vigorously they're probably thrusting.

Instead, armed with the knowledge that you're excited about strap-on play, grab a sex-ed book on the topic or a how-to video that's meant to be educational and head to your local sex-positive sex-toy store for advice and supplies. And when you try it yourself, start incredibly slow. Just remember, porn is for mining ideas and getting turned on, not for learning how to do new things.

For some people, porn is distracting. No matter how well made, they can't get past the settings, or the dialogue, or maybe they're just not attracted to the performers. Never fear! That's where written erotica comes in.

The great thing about erotic literature is that your mind can fill in lots of details such that it fits your taste more than sex on film might. Sure, the author likely describes the characters to you somewhat, but there's still lots of room for interpretation. The resources section also has suggestions for where to start if you want to read erotica. (And shameless self-promotion time—I've written some you can find, too.)

With erotica, I suggest starting with anthologies. A book of short stories gives you lots of chances to find something you like rather than trying to slog through a whole novel that isn't to your taste. Some anthologies will be centered on a theme, like bondage, and some run the gamut of topics.

There are even anthologies of short shorts, where stories are only five hundred or a thousand words. How simple is that? In less than five minutes, you can read a whole story and see if the topic, or acts involved, appeal to you. And because they're so short, you can give several a try. Leave room for a particular author's voice not being to your style, rather than immediately assuming you're not into the things they're describing.

But like the exercises above where you write things down from your own fantasies or memories, erotic stories give you concrete examples of ways people can have sex or kink play that you can take for a test-drive in the fantasy realm before you try the real thing.

As you're reading, pay close attention to what turns you on. Maybe it's the acts people are engaging in or maybe it's the power dynamics. Maybe the terms people are calling each other are getting your attention, or maybe there's something about the setting that turns you on.

For your first read through, just mark the pages of the stories that turn you on. Then you can go back for a second, or third, more critical reading. What exactly was it that worked for you? You can keep a separate page of notes where you track the elements you like and how you'd like to incorporate them into your life.

You and your partner can also read erotica out loud to each other as a bedtime story, or as part of foreplay. You can do this for the same reasons as above, to get turned on and discover things you might like, or you can also use erotica to bring fantasies into the bedroom that you like in theory but prefer stay on the page. More on that later.

YOUR WANT LIST

It can be really useful to have a short list of things you know you like in mind at all times. Whether you're having a one-night stand, an adventure at a play party, or even a night with your main squeeze, having a few things in mind keeps you from freezing up when you're on the spot.

Some folks do this for food—they know what their two or three go-to recipes are, so when they're tired, hungry, or have unexpected guests they don't have to think too hard about what's for dinner. And just because something is your easy fallback doesn't mean it isn't also a favorite. Pizza might be an easy dinner choice, but people are rarely disappointed when a pizza shows up.

So what is your pizza of sex?

If someone approached you at a play party, or your partner asked you what would feel good after a long day, what would you ask for without having to think about it too much?

For me, I'm pretty much always happy to receive a foot rub. A back rub is also acceptable. Snuggling and watching a movie or snuggling up while someone reads to me are also favorites. I know I'm going to enjoy these things without having to spend any time thinking about what I want.

Not every date is the right time for adventures that require supplies and setup. It helps to have a go-to routine that's satisfying for everyone but doesn't feel daunting to get ready for.

You can also have a favorite sex toy that's your go-to choice for pizza-night sex. Maybe it's something you use with a partner and maybe it's something you use alone. Mutual masturbation is another option that can be an easy way to connect, relax, and even get off without feeling like you need to muster extra energy.

No matter how simple or involved your list of favorites is, try to keep the supplies you need for them on hand, the way you'd keep staples in the pantry, so that you're always ready to go. Lube is one of those basic supplies that should always be handy. Maybe a favorite vibrator or sex toy is, too. Your safer-sex supplies of choice should also be within reach at all times. These aren't things you want to go out of your way to think about—you want them handy right when you need them.

YOUR MAYBE-LATER LIST

On my adventures through sex and kink events, I've seen a lot of different kinds of play. One of the things I love about parties is all the ideas I get from them. And even when I see things I might not want to do right then, I love knowing that there will never be a shortage of new things to try. Similar to the yes/no/maybe list, you can keep a maybe-later list of things you might want to revisit in a few months, or even a few years.

You can add to this list whenever you see something in a book, a movie, or at an event. You can add to it whenever you stumble upon a new fantasy or have a sexy dream. The great thing about it being the maybe-later list is that there's no rush or pressure to try these things. In fact, you might never get to them. And the list can be private if you'd like, or you can share it with a partner or partners. Whatever makes you feel most comfortable.

This list can be a great way to track things that have caught your eye, but for whatever reason don't seem like a great idea right now. And not only can you use the list to get ideas for future play, or for things you might want to learn about, but over time you might notice trends on your list.

Like any of the other fantasy exploration exercises we've discussed, this list can be a place where you start to notice themes or patterns among the things that are catching your eye. Even if you never try any of the exact items on your list, you might gain some valuable insight about your desires and find ways to incorporate the same themes in different ways that feel safer or more comfortable right now.

NOW WHAT?

If you've been doing all the exercises in this chapter, you've probably made an impressive dent in your notebook. That's great! Keep everything you've done handy, and be ready to keep adding to it. This will be a living document for you as your interests, desires, and partners change over time. The information you've uncovered about yourself will also serve you well as you dive into the hands-on exercises, and now that you've done this work to discover what you want, the next chapter will help you talk to your partner(s) about it.

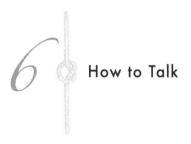

How to Talk

INTRO TO TALKING

ONCE YOU'RE READY TO SIT DOWN WITH A partner and talk about sex, or start incorporating more chat into the sex you're having—how do you start? If you're wondering what talking would look like and what specific tools you can use, this is the chapter for you. We're going to cover everything from styles of communication to listening skills to hands-on exercises you can try in the bedroom.

There's a lot of information here, and it can be easy to get overwhelmed. Give yourself permission to read one section at a time, or to take breaks as needed. And when you're ready, take notes on two or three things you'll try incorporating into your conversations or your sex the next chance you get.

You don't need to overhaul everything all at once. Sometimes just a few little changes to the language you're using can make a huge difference in results. There are enough tools here that if the first couple you try don't work for you, there are plenty more to try. As you work your way through, you'll get a feeling for your style of communication and which techniques are most likely to work for you.

Keep in mind that many of the things in life worth doing are scary, and even if this feels hard at first, the payoff will be well worth it. But don't forget that you get to move at your own pace, so don't feel pressure to try a lot of new things right away. The whole point is your pleasure, and you're the only one who can decide what's right for you.

BODY-PART WORDS

Before we look at how to start these conversations, let's talk about the language we use to describe bodies. What language do you like used around your body? What terms do you use for your chest, or for your genitals?

When I teach my class Mapping the Vulva, I start by asking people to tell me their favorite terms for this body part, followed by their least favorite terms, while I write them on a whiteboard. Every time, at least one word ends up on both the favorite and least favorite list. And every time, I've got a great example of the point I want to make.

Once again, what seems obvious to one person isn't really obvious at all. And when it comes to language around bodies, there is a huge amount of variation. I spent years as an erotica writer and ended up reading a wide range of stories as I was going through the books in which my stories appeared. One thing became incredibly clear to me: if an author used body-part words I didn't like, the whole story was ruined for me.

This is doubly true when you're in the bedroom with

someone. Few things ruin the mood faster than someone using a word about your body that doesn't resonate with you. It can be anything from a turnoff to a trigger. And it's so easy to add this point to your sexual negotiation. Simply ask someone what words they like to use around their body. Or, if you must, just wait and mirror the language that the person uses about themselves.

Another way to start the conversation is to try to use words that seem generic, while you wait to ask for preferred terms. Although it might sound clinical, you could use the word *genitals* (I've also heard that shortened into a cute nickname, gennies). Other generic words like *parts, bits,* or even *junk* can work. Having an awareness of your vocabulary will give you a great foundation from which to hold all sorts of conversations.

OPEN-ENDED QUESTIONS

In just about every class I teach, at some point I encourage people to move past asking, "Is this okay?" I'm not talking about checking for consent—that's mandatory. But assuming you're already participating in consensual activities, you want to use your check-ins to help you build an optimal experience.

If the person you're asking likes you, and the thing you're doing isn't horrible, the answer to "Is this okay?" is almost always yes. And while making sure what you're doing isn't horrible is a great start, most of us would like to do much better than that.

It can be tricky, because people who aren't used to talking about sex or asking for what they want might not have all the language for their desires at first. But it's a skill that's worth building.

Instead of asking yes or no questions, asking open-ended questions can be a powerful communication technique. Your partner is likely to give you a lot more information than you'd otherwise get. Here are some questions to get you started:

- How do you like to be touched?
- What would make this better?

If completely open-ended questions seem like too much, try starting with a choice between options:
-
- Harder or softer
- Faster or slower
- Left or right

Wondering how that could look in action? Imagine this scenario: you're with a new partner and you're still learning their body. You've already negotiated for sexual play and you're in bed together, exploring each other's bodies. The clothes have come off, you've spent a while kissing, and after stroking her thighs for a while, as her hips buck toward your hand, you ask if you can take her panties off. She says yes. You've already talked about what kind of language to use around each other's bodies, and you know she prefers the term *vulva,* so you ask if you can touch her vulva. She says yes again. You ask how she likes to be touched. And then . . . her mouth opens, but she doesn't answer. She's never been asked that question before and isn't sure what to say.

"Let's try this," you say, and you begin touching her. You start by placing your whole hand over her vulva, so she can get used to being touched. As she relaxes you begin to stroke her labia. As she relaxes into that and her legs fall open more comfortably, you start gently stroking her clit. After doing that for a couple of minutes you feel her body moving in rhythm with your hand. "Would you like me to stroke you harder or softer?" you ask.

"Harder," she says, and you increase the pressure you're using to touch her.

Her breathing is becoming unsteady and she's moaning softly between intakes of breath. Her hips are pressing up toward your hand more insistently. "Do you want me to speed up?" you ask, and she says, "Yes, faster."

Are you starting to get the idea how you might integrate these questions into your sex life? It doesn't have to be the stilted, awkward interruptions most people imagine when I suggest they talk during sex. It can be sexy. It can be part of dirty talk. And it can help you have better sex. Maybe even amazing sex.

Another useful tool can be scaling questions. If you've ever been to the hospital, you've probably been asked to rate your pain on a scale from one to ten. You've also probably encountered this if you've explored kinky play. Well, scaling questions can be used for pleasure, too. If you ask how good something feels on a scale of one to ten, and then modify what you're doing and ask again, you've got a concrete data point about whether the changes made things better or worse. You can even repurpose the children's game where you ask if you're getting warmer or colder, to find the hidden treat in the room.

These types of games and questions are great for people who aren't used to talking about pleasure, or who don't yet know what to ask for. They also lend themselves to playfulness and exploration, which is a great tone to set when you're experimenting with what kinds of touch you and your partner(s) might enjoy.

Open-ended questions aren't just helpful during sex or when talking about touch. They're also great for asking about your partner's fantasies or for asking about their concerns about a situation, sexual or otherwise.

Saying, "I'm curious about rope bondage, would you like to try it with me?" is a wonderful and direct way to see if a partner is willing to try something you're interested in. But that won't help you figure out desires they haven't mentioned yet.

Try something like, "How about I tell you one of my fantasies, and then you share one of yours?" And that's just one way to get the conversation started. By offering to go first, you're making yourself vulnerable, and that in turn may make your partner feel safer being vulnerable.

When you're using open-ended questions for nonsexual talk, here are a few you can try:

- ▸ "What would make you feel heard?"
- ▸ "What would make you feel listened to?"
- ▸ "What would make you feel understood?"

As you can see, open-ended questions in or out of the bedroom give people a platform to communicate about their needs and getting those needs met. There's a learning curve, but once you get used to this style of communication, it becomes second nature.

THE POWER OF CHANGING YOUR MIND

Have you ever been to an ice cream shop that's known for its outrageous flavors? Everything from garlic to bone marrow to squid ink seems to be having its culinary moment. And while that might pique your interest, you probably don't want to dive right into a whole scoop. That's why ice cream shops offer you those little taster spoons. You can find out what flavors you like, or what you're in the mood for that day, without making a big commitment.

The same is true of sex or kink. To find out all the things you might enjoy, you've got to be free to give something a little taste to decide if you like it, and tasting isn't a commitment to have any more.

The problem is, when it comes to sex, we tend to have a more all-or-nothing attitude than when it comes to ice cream. If people try something and don't like it, sometimes one or both people won't speak up for fear that will end the whole encounter.

That's where the power of changing your mind comes in. Try something, and if you don't like it, try something else! It's not the end of the play, just the end of that particular act.

Here's how that could go in your bedroom:

Plan in advance for a particular evening to be about experimenting. Have something new you'd like to try (or even a couple of things) and talk in advance about how you'd like that to go. Talk about everything from learning to do the thing to doing the thing safely. You can also set a time limit, or just plan to have open communication and lots of check-ins.

Make sure it's clear that this is no more high risk than trying an ice cream flavor. If you don't like it, that's fine. There are dozens more flavors to try, and there's no shame in falling back on one of your all-time favorites. So if you try spanking and aren't into it? Fine! You still get to have the kind of play or sex you usually enjoy. Stopping the spanking doesn't mean all play has to stop (unless you want it to).

Try to institute this policy on a full-time basis. Any activity that's introduced with "Hey, would you like to try . . ." implies that it's just an ice cream taster spoon-size attempt. That way you get in the habit of not being penalized for changing your mind, and it gets easier and easier to do.

"I" STATEMENTS

There are several schools of thought about how to have the most productive conversations and how to make your-self heard without activating defensiveness in the person listening.

One way to have productive conversations is to use "I" statements. Framing feedback this way can be helpful to own your feelings, wants, and needs. Starting a statement with "I" can help you be listened to and heard, rather than the other person shutting down or taking a defensive stance. Imagine these two conversations starters:

"You're not listening to me—put your phone down when I'm talking."

"I feel like I'm not being heard right now. Do I have your full attention?"

Using "I" statements can also help you avoid coming across as passive or indirect. Try saying, "I feel ready to move in together, can we talk about that?" rather than saying, "Bob and Sally just got a house . . ." and hoping the other person will read between the lines.

"I" statements are often formulated as a way to avoid "you" statements, or statements that could be read as an accusation. When we accuse someone of something, they take a defensive stance. When we state our feelings, we're more likely to be met with empathy.

How might this look when it comes to sex and romance? Maybe you're feeling insecure, or unwanted, and in frustration you accuse your partner, "You're not attracted to me anymore." That statement isn't likely to lead to a productive conversation. Instead try, "I'm feeling insecure and could use some reassurance. Can you give me some compliments?"

You may have noticed from previous examples that "I" statements often take the form of sharing feelings, and that's one of the ways they're the most effective. Even when someone is yelling at their partner for getting home late, what's underneath that is a feeling of hurt or frustration. And while none of us will ever be perfect at this, learning to lead conversations by telling our partner how we're feeling is likely to be more effective than simply lashing out.

STAY POSITIVE

Along with avoiding assumptions, staying positive is a theme in this book. That's because it comes up again and again with clients and students. It's important to remember that just because there's something you want to work on, it doesn't mean everything is terrible. And it can help to frame the conversation with what's already working, or in a positive light.

I hear from people that they're afraid to ask for a new kind of sex, or a modification to the sex they're already having, because they're afraid their partner will interpret that to mean that all the current things they're doing are lousy. But that's rarely what people mean, and you can head off that assumption by adjusting your language.

One way of doing this is "sandwiching," where you make a positive statement before and after the thing that needs improvement. So, you could say, "I really love the way you touch me. It would help me reach orgasm if we incorporated sex toys into our play. I'm excited by the idea of expanding our intimacy in that way." By leading with something positive (as long as it's true), you can head off hurt feelings or bruised egos, or the chance of derailing the conversation because the other person assumes everything is awful.

You can also just lead with a positive, like, "This feels amazing and I think it could be even better if we tried it in another position." This way when you're asking for a change, you make it absolutely clear it's not because you don't enjoy what's happening, you just think there's room for improvement.

Another tool that I sneaked into the example above is saying "and" where it might have felt more natural to say "but." Saying "but" can feel like it's negating what was said already, whereas "and" simply adds to it.

See how it feels in this example: "I love you, but I get

frustrated when a week goes by without having sex." In that sentence it can feel like the "but" is saying that the love is somehow impacted by the time without sex. Which can make someone feel like the love will be lost if sex doesn't happen.

Here's the sentence again with that one word changed: "I love you, and I get frustrated when a week goes by without having sex." In this instance, the "and" makes it clear that those two things can both be true at once. Even when there's frustration about sex, there's still love.

In that example, you can see how vital that one change can be. It might seem small, swapping one three-letter word for another, but words are powerful things, and even a small change in the language we use can have a big impact.

DESIRE + BOUNDARY

For some people, setting boundaries can seem difficult. One way to clearly establish a boundary is by coupling it with the request that you're making. So you could say something like, "I'd love a massage, but only on my neck and shoulders," or "I'd love to snuggle for a while, but let's keep our clothes on." That way you've both established an activity that you'd like to do and stated a boundary about how far you'd like that activity to go.

LISTENING SKILLS

A huge part of communicating is listening, but I think sometimes we miss this piece. When people tell you they're a good communicator, they usually mean that they think they speak clearly. That their meaning is understood. But that's one-way communication.

The kind of communication we need in relationships must go both ways. We need to fully hear and understand what our partners are telling us and respond to what is really being shared, not just the version our mind interprets.

At some point you've probably heard of, or even practiced, active listening skills. It's a way to fully engage with what is being said to you, rather than waiting for your turn to speak or thinking of what you're going to say next.

This is easier said than done when emotions are involved. When a partner brings up a problem or a touchy subject, or even just makes a request, we often jump to wondering what this means about us. It's natural to get defensive, or to feel hurt or inadequate. That's because when it comes to sex and relationships, we're filtering everything we hear through our own perceptions, and some of us are likely to hear the worst possible version of what's being said to us.

But when we go to that mental space, when we make what our partner is saying about us, we aren't really hearing them. We aren't able to engage with what they're saying in a way that will lead to a useful outcome. Sometimes this means we need to hear what our partner has to say and then take a break to process our feelings before coming back to respond.

If you're one of the people who hears the worst version of what's being said, and your partner says they'd like to try a new kind of sex, you might jump to the conclusion that your partner is bored with you or thinks you're bad at sex. And those fears and feelings run so deep, it's easy to respond in a way that turns the discussion into an argument, or at least shuts down the conversation. When a request from your partner goes that way, there's a chance they'll never risk bringing up that kind of topic again. And then you miss out on knowing what would turn your partner on, or on getting to try new and exciting things.

Here are some ways to listen and to make sure you're hearing what's being said:

- ▸ Ask clarifying questions
  - ▹ Not only does this help make sure you really understand what's being said, but it helps the other person feel heard.
- ▸ Reflect what you're hearing and let the other person explain if it's not what they meant
  - ▹ Keep in mind that this can become irritating if done too often, or if it sounds like you're mocking your partner by repeating them, so use this tactic carefully.
- ▸ Ask if the person just wants to be heard or if they want help brainstorming solutions
  - ▹ Few things irritate people more than having someone offer solutions when all they wanted was a sympathetic shoulder to cry on.

When listening to our partners, sometimes we need to listen between the lines a bit. That's not to give people a free pass, allowing them not to communicate clearly—it's simply an acknowledgment that when talking about vulnerable topics, we don't always have all the right words right away.

If and when you have the bandwidth to do it, consider

this—the next time a partner seems angry, or like they're accusing you of something, try saying, "I hear that you're really frustrated right now . . ." When someone hears that what they're feeling is being acknowledged, it can sometimes move the conversation in a more productive direction.

LISTENING WITHOUT JUDGMENT

When your partner opens up to you about a fantasy they have, you can bet it was a big deal for them to do so. Even if what they want isn't something you're into, it's important to listen without judgment. Being shamed for our desires can cause deep scars, and if your partner learns it isn't safe to share with you, you can bet you won't hear about their other fantasies.

Try to keep a neutral face and just listen. Hear everything they have to say and give yourself a moment to think about it. If you're not ready to answer right away, it's okay to ask for more time. But whatever you do, don't freak out about what they've suggested.

If a partner reveals something personal about their desires, here are some ways you could respond:

- ▸ "I really appreciate the vulnerability it took to share that with me."
- ▸ "I appreciate you trusting me with that."
- ▸ "I'm so glad you feel comfortable sharing with me."
- ▸ "Thank you for telling me."

Of course, the person who has just opened up will also be waiting to hear what you think of the idea, and if it's something you want to engage in. If you're not up for it, here are some things you can follow up with:

▸ "I don't think there's anything wrong with that, but it isn't my cup of tea."

▸ "It doesn't bother me if you do that, but I don't want to participate."

▸ "I don't think that's for me, but I'm glad you told me about it. I love you."

You'll be better able to listen without judgment if you've gone through the exercises in chapter 2 about working through your biases. Because it's almost certain that a partner will be into something you're not into at some point in your life, and we don't want to leave people with shame scars just for having different turn-ons.

SAYING OR HEARING NO

I'm excited when someone says no to me, because it means if/when that person says yes to something, I can believe them. Being able to trust that someone can and will say no means that I can try more adventurous things and know that the other person is doing them because they really want to, and not because they're trying to please me.

Imagine this: you're dating someone and whenever you suggest a restaurant or a movie they just say, "Sure," and go along with whatever you want. Does there come a point when you wonder if they really just have the same exact taste in food and movies as you do or if, more likely, they're just trying to be easygoing?

When you go home with that person and want to suggest a new kind of sex, and they still say, "Sure," would you be second-guessing if they were really into it? I certainly would. In fact, I probably wouldn't even be having sex with that person. I want a demonstrated history of someone speaking up for themselves before I try anything remotely risky or vulnerable with them.

In kink circles this is often summed up as "If you can't trust someone's no, you can't trust their yes." Issues like this become especially important in kink, because the risks are a lot higher than simply choosing what's for dinner. So it's important that everyone involved has gotten really comfortable saying no to things.

And if you're a maybe? Say that, too. But when it comes to sex and kink, a maybe is a no. Or at least a no for now. It can mean that you'll spend more time talking about it, or researching the topic, but don't try something new until you're an unreserved yes about it.

What happens when you've done the self-work and exploration to figure out what it is you desire, you work up the guts to ask your partner, and then they say no? First of all, remember that hearing no can be a good thing. You know that your partner is able to set boundaries, and that means it's safe to ask them about new things. But that doesn't mean it isn't hard to hear.

You can always go with the classic "thank you for taking care of yourself," because we always want to honor people for setting boundaries.

WHERE IS YOUR PARTNER COMING FROM?

Different cultures, different religions, and different families have very different takes on sex and sexuality. Learning about where your partner comes from can help you understand where they are now.

If someone was raised being told that masturbation is

wrong or a sin, that can explain why they might not know everything about how their body likes to be touched, or might be uncomfortable with you watching them touch themselves.

Asking questions about people's early sex education can be a great way to start understanding how your partner ticks when it comes to sex. Once you've broached the subject and your partner has agreed to have this conversation, here are some questions you can ask:

▶ When did you first get "the talk"? Who did it come from and what did it include?

▶ Did you have sex ed in school? If so, do you remember at what age and what was included?

▶ How did your parents/family talk about dating and relationships?

▶ How did your parents/family talk about sex? (If at all.)

▶ Were you a part of any religious organizations that shared information about sex or sexuality? If so, what were those messages?

▶ What were your early sexual experiences with your own body like? When did you start exploring?

▶ How has your upbringing affected how you currently feel about sex and dating?

▶ Do you remember getting specific negative messages about anything to do with sex, sexuality, kink, or relationships?

▶ Was nonsexual touch a regular part of your childhood? Hugs, snuggles, etc.?

▶ Were the adults in your household affectionate with each other?

▸ Were spanking or other forms of physical punishment used?

▸ What messages did you hear about people's motivations for sex?

▸ What gender-based assumptions or stereotypes did you see/hear?

These questions only scratch the surface, but they can begin to paint a picture of someone's upbringing and the stories around sex they might carry with them today.

Just as important can be to spend some time thinking about where your beliefs around sex, sexuality, and relationships came from. You can answer these questions for yourself, in conversation with your partner, or as prompts for a journaling exercise.

However you decide to tackle your sexual background, and that of your partner(s), you might be surprised how many of these early messages are still with you and still affecting your sex life.

LESSONS FROM BUSINESS

What can we learn from our professional communication to apply to our personal life? More than you might expect. Even people who consider themselves good communicators run into trouble in sexual or romantic relationships. Why? Because we make more assumptions than in other forms of communication.

One way to improve your communication is to take the skills you have already (and maybe don't even realize you have) and start applying them to your relationships.

When people send an email for business, they tend to be very concise and clear. Why are you writing? What do you want? What happens next? We don't expect our business associates to read our minds the way we sometimes expect our partners to. So what would happen if you approached intimate communication the way you approach business communication?

> ‣ You'd state the purpose of your communication.
> ‣ You'd ask about the best time/way to talk.
> ‣ You'd be explicit about follow-up.

Let's break those down and apply them to our intimate lives.

State the purpose of your communication. If you're writing to a vendor for your business to get quotes on pamphlets or postcards, you'd say so in the subject line of your email. So when you want to bring up a sensitive topic with a partner, try saying what you want to talk about right up front: "Hey, honey, I'd love to talk to you about having our first threesome."

Next up, in a professional email, you generally ask if they prefer phone/Skype/email and when the best time to talk would be. The same goes for sensitive talks with a partner. Some people like to have tricky conversations at home, and others would rather do it in public. Some people like having relationship talks via email, when they can get all their thoughts down without the pressure of face-to-face interaction, and other people find written communication too impersonal for intimate discussions.

Taking our lesson from business, we'd ask about the best way to talk: "Can we talk about threesomes over dinner tonight? Or would you rather save it for the weekend?"

Finally, be clear about what comes next. Do you think a resolution has been reached? Say so explicitly. Is it something you need to think about? Say that, too. And also set a time when you'll check back in on this topic.

It's amazing but true that two people in a conversation can take different things out of it. So especially if the conversation is high stakes, make absolutely sure you both got the same thing out of it. In a business email, you'll often reflect the understanding that has been reached.

It's also not a terrible idea to put things in writing. Have a little journal for relationship discussions and boundaries that you both/all have access to so you can refer back to any decisions or agreements that have been made: "I'm so glad we finally talked about this! I'll think about which of my friends I'd like to approach, while you do the same, and we'll check back in about this next Friday."

Maybe you think I'm overstating the chances of miscommunication, but I've heard stories where someone expresses a passing interest in threesomes, or at least a willingness to talk about them, only to have their partner show up with a third on their next date. This is a surefire way to get one or more people's feelings hurt—or to have someone pressured into something they'll regret later.

You've got other business skills I bet you haven't thought of using for a relationship, too. Have you ever negotiated a salary for a new job or a raise at your current gig? Then you might be familiar with the idea of asking for the salary you really want first, but knowing what the minimum you'll accept is.

In business, as in sex and relationships, it's helpful to know what we want and need in advance of conversations, so we don't feel rushed to make a snap decision or pressured to compromise on something that really won't work for us.

With sex and relationships, sometimes there's wiggle room in what will work for us, and sometimes there isn't. I'm not suggesting you compromise on anything that is essential to your happiness and well-being. But with some fantasies and interests, there's a range of outcomes we could be happy with.

Say you have a fantasy about having public sex while you're blindfolded and tied up and you know people are watching you. That could be your dream scenario. But maybe there are privacy concerns that make that impractical for you or your partner, or maybe your partner just isn't into it.

So what would it take for you to still feel like you're getting to scratch that itch? Maybe it's trying bondage and a blindfold at home, but without the audience. Maybe it's going to a public club, but playing in a private room. Maybe it's blindfolding you and then using dirty talk to describe an imaginary audience that's watching you naked and tied up. This can be a great way to get creative about the different ways to experience things that excite us.

TALKING ABOUT SPEED AND PACING

By this point you've probably got the idea that people should check in before moving to new activities, and also have an idea of what activities are on the table for any given encounter. But even with this level of communication taken care of, there are some subtleties that can be missed.

If you don't want to be the kid in the back seat on a road trip asking, "Are we there yet?" every five minutes, it's a good idea to talk about the pace at which you'd like to move. Some people want to stick with kissing and making out for a long time before moving to other things, and other people are used to ripping off garments as soon as the door is closed.

Neither of these approaches are wrong, but those two people could be a mismatch for each other if they can't negotiate and find a pace that works well for both of them. Just like stating any other sexual preferences, you can come right out and say, "I like to spend a long time kissing before we move on to other things." This makes it clear to the other person where you're coming from, and they're not left wondering what's up when you're not advancing things they way they expected, and you don't have to slow them down or move their hand every five minutes.

For folks who like to get naked right away? It's okay to say that, too: "Hey, I wanted to let you know that I like getting clothes off ASAP. Doesn't mean I want to rush through sex—I just like enjoying the whole buffet at once." Again, this lets the other person know where you're coming from, and it gives them a chance to speak up if it's not their style. Otherwise you might find yourself entirely undressed while the other person hasn't even taken their shoes off.

COMFORT WITH BEING NAKED

What helps you feel most comfortable with a partner? Not everyone likes being seen naked. Some people prefer sex with the lights out or under the covers. Some people go to the bathroom to change into pajamas or a nightgown.

Wherever your comfort level is, that's fine. But if you do want to be naked with a partner, what would help make that feel great?

Sometimes starting with nonsexual nudity is the way to go. If there's a nude beach or nude hot-tubbing place in your area, those can both be great options for raising your comfort level with nudity. Maybe you think being naked with strangers sounds even worse, but hear me out. In spaces that allow nonsexual nudity, people usually aren't checking each other out. Many of these spaces even have explicit rules against it, or maybe they're framed as "don't be creepy."

In Portland, where I live, there are even children present at all of these places, and that really helps set the tone as firmly nonsexual. What that means is that you have a space where you can start to get used to nakedness not being a big deal. Sure, there can be a sensual pleasure to feeling water or sun or sand on your body. But it isn't about sex. It's just about enjoying being in your skin. And that's the perfect place to start if you're feeling concerned about how your body looks. Try shifting the focus to how your body can feel and what your body can do.

If you go to a space like this with your partner, you'll also be able to practice being naked together, but not touching. Some of these places allow no touch whatsoever, and some will allow casual touch like holding hands. Either way, it can help enforce the idea that just because there's nudity, there doesn't have to be sex.

America has an especially complicated view when it comes to bodies, nudity, and sex. In plenty of other countries and cultures, things like spas and bathhouses and beaches are regularly enjoyed nude, by the whole family.

And you know what? Those cultures are often more comfortable with their bodies.

But many of us have been raised to see nudity, and bodies, as shameful. And that feeling can get in the way of being able to enjoy sex. Having sex under the covers or with the lights out is possible, but it poses more of a logistical challenge. If you're not adjusting your movements to keep the covers on and you have enough light to see what you're doing, it'll make certain kinds of sex a lot easier. That doesn't mean you need to erect stadium lights in your bedroom. Even a red lightbulb or a few candles will do the trick. But it helps to be able to see what you're doing so you don't accidentally land an elbow in someone's face.

If public places are out of the question, you can also warm up to nudity in your own space with just your partner. Sometimes taking a shower together is a great way to start, because it's a place where many of us already feel comfortable naked. When you shower with a partner (even if you've explicitly stated this isn't for sex), there can be ways you explore touching each other's bodies that can feel easier, because there's a purpose or a road map.

When it comes time for sexual touch, sometimes we feel lost or unsure what to do, but most of us are pretty clear on how to wash our bodies. So maybe you start with washing each other's backs in the shower. This can help build familiarity with each other's bodies in a place where there's no pressure to move to sex.

Another way to build comfort around bodies and nudity is to exchange compliments. When doing so, it's important to know what kind of language we like used around our bodies. Sometimes people give compliments they think we'll enjoy, but really they become turnoffs or make us feel bad about ourselves.

This came up with a recent podcast question that I was called in to answer. A woman in her forties started dating men in their twenties after a long-term relationship ended. She was finding a trend of these men saying things like "I love your fat ass," or "you're so thick," and she knew they meant them nicely, but once those words were out, she felt incredibly self-conscious and couldn't enjoy herself.

Ultimately this was a problem of language. These guys were trying to give compliments, and it seemed like they genuinely thought the terms they were using were flattering. Maybe it was a generational shift, but for whatever reason, the giver and the receiver of the compliments were speaking different languages.

Luckily, this is an easy problem to solve. You can either warn someone before clothes have ever come off what kinds of language you find flattering and what you don't like, or you can offer a correction after something you don't like. In a situation like this, you could say, "I know you're trying to compliment me and I really appreciate that, and also the words you're using make me uncomfortable. Instead of saying 'fat' or 'thick,' could you say you love my curves?" Or if commenting on body specifics is still too much, you could say, "I'm glad you enjoy my body. It would help me stay in the moment if you didn't say anything that refers to size or specifics, and instead just tell me that I'm beautiful." Whatever is true for you, it's always okay to negotiate for the kind of language you want used around your body, just as you would negotiate for the kinds of touch or sex acts you're comfortable with.

TIEBREAKERS

I was in law school with an adorable couple (who had adorable dogs), and they had some wonderful systems for managing communication in their relationship. One technique they had that I'll never forget was using the scaling system not for pain or for pleasure, but for how much they wanted something. For example, if they were deciding what to have for dinner, maybe one would want Thai food and the other would want Mexican. Inevitably they'd move to the scaling question:

"How much do you want Thai food?"

"I want it about a five. How much do you want Mexican food?"

"Been thinking about it all day, I'm like an eight."

And that's how they'd decide. Whoever felt stronger about the thing would win. I don't think that system would work for everyone, but within their relationship they'd come up with a technique for breaking a tie. Of course, this system requires honesty and not fudging to get your way. And for that to work, you already have to be happy with your partner and be in a fairly good place.

The other useful technique they had was that if someone turned down a suggestion, that person had to make the next suggestion. So, to use the Thai versus Mexican example, it might go something like this:

"Do you feel like Thai food tonight?"

"No."

"Okay, what do you want?"

"How about Mexican food?"

That way, the work to make a decision is equally on both people, rather than one person making suggestions and the other knocking them down one by one.

These techniques can work for sexual communication, too. Now, I'm not suggesting you pressure or coerce someone into sex when they don't feel like it. But sometimes it's more a matter of indecision rather than disinterest. Some of this problem can be solved by defining your terms, as we discussed in chapter 3, but sometimes it's helpful to use the counteroffer method described above. How would that work for sex? Maybe something like this:

"Do you feel like having sex tonight?"

"Not really."

"Is there another way we could be intimate with each other?"

"How about taking a shower together and then masturbating next to each other?"

Just like deciding what to have for dinner, the person who said no to the first offer makes the next suggestion. And although I said this above, I want to emphasize again—"no" is always an acceptable answer and a complete sentence. These techniques are only for when both parties really do want to find a way to engage with each other.

COMPLIMENTS AND GRATITUDE

Talking to your partner(s) isn't just for when you want something to change. It's important to make expressing compliments and gratitude a regular part of your routine, too. Tell someone they look good when you see them for a date. Tell them when you like the way they're touching you. Tell them you're proud when they've achieved a goal or milestone they've been working toward.

Not only is this just basic support and niceness, but

it's important to have a solid foundation before you start trying new or challenging things. If you've never said anything that you like or enjoy and then start talking about something you'd like to change, it might not be received well.

Compliments are also a great way to let our partners know what's working for us. Just like telling someone you like their outfit makes it more likely they'll wear it around you again, telling someone you like the way they're touching you makes it more likely they'll do that again, too.

Try to get into the habit of commenting on things you appreciate, because too many things are taken for granted. You probably like things about your partner that it's never occurred to you to say out loud. Try to be mindful and aware during your interactions so that you can notice, and comment on, all the things you appreciate and enjoy.

General compliments can be lovely, but specific compliments are sometimes more meaningful. You can (and should) still tell someone they're beautiful, handsome, lovely, or sexy, but also let them know exactly what you like. The way their skin looks? They way they smell? Most of us have things we're attracted to that other people might never consider, like the slope of a neck or a forearm disappearing into a rolled-up sleeve.

QUESTIONS TO ASK WHEN TRYING SOMETHING NEW

Whenever you're planning to try something new, it's important to have a conversation about it first. The more different the activity is from your usual play, the more you're going to want to talk about it first. And as we've established, there can be a variety of reasons people want to engage in any given activity.

Not only that, but trying new things can be scary. And those fears can be reasons we haven't tried the new thing sooner, or maybe why we're afraid to try it now. When you talk openly with your partner(s) about what the concerns are, you're able to address them together. Sometimes it's a simple matter of reassurances, or sometimes there are concrete steps you can take—like making sure you learn to do the new thing safely.

So in order to set yourself up for success, it's helpful to talk about your motivations, and your fears, before you get started. Here are some questions you can ask yourself and discuss with your partner:

> ‣ What are you hoping to get from this new experience?
> ‣ What scares you about this new experience?
> ‣ What turns you on about the idea of this new experience?

If you're wondering what that would look like in practice, here's how trying bondage for the first time could go.

What are you hoping to get from this new experience?

> ‣ You want to play with vulnerability between you and your partner, either one way or taking turns. You're using bondage as a way to let one person be vulnerable to the other, and to play with and experience trust.
> ‣ One of you has a hard time relaxing and receiving pleasure, so you're using bondage as a way to help

that person get used to simply receiving sensation without immediately trying to reciprocate.

▸ You're curious about BDSM or dominance and submission and you're using bondage as a way to explore.

▸ You're having a hard time focusing on intimacy, so you're using shibari (Japanese bondage) as a way to spend more time with each other's bodies, as the rope gives you a road map of where to touch.

▸ You want to spice things up a little and do something that feels taboo, so you're taking a rope-bondage class together.

What scares you about this new experience?

▸ You're afraid the rope will be uncomfortable, or that you'll get hurt.

▸ You're afraid you won't like bondage, and that will disappoint your partner.

▸ You're afraid you won't be good at learning the knots, and that will be disappointing or embarrassing.

▸ You're afraid that if you start trying kink, "regular sex" will feel boring.

What turns you on about the idea of this new experience?

▸ You like the sensual feeling of rope against your skin.

▸ You're turned on by the vulnerability and the restricted movement.

▸ You like the idea of giving up control.

▸ You like having focused attention on your body.

Once you've each explored all of these questions, you're not only ready to try something new and exciting, but you're setting yourself up for the best chance of a good experience.

POSTPLAY DEBRIEFING

One of the best ways you can figure out what you like is to try lots of things. Then use what you've learned from those experiments to have an even better experience the next time you play. So how do you learn from an experience in a way that helps you grow and advance your skills? Communication, of course! This time in the form of a postplay debriefing. These conversations are more common in kink but are valuable for everyone no matter what kind of sex or play you're having.

You don't want to launch into this conversation while you're still in the middle of afterglow. Wait a few days after you've played so that you have time to really think about what happened. It might help to keep a journal for yourself so you can note how you felt about everything, what you liked best, and where there was room for improvement.

When you know how you feel about what happened, then it's time to talk to your partner(s) about it. Like with other conversations we've discussed, make sure everyone involved opts in to having the debriefing talk—don't surprise someone with it. This also gives everyone time to think about the experience before the conversation happens.

When you have your talk, start with the positive:

- ▶ "I love that we tried something new."
- ▶ "I like how you touched me."
- ▶ "I felt really safe."

▶ "I appreciated your vulnerability."
▶ "I had a wonderful orgasm."
▶ "I love that it was playful, and we could laugh together."

Next, talk about what didn't really work for you. Think about things that you wouldn't want to do again, or things that could be improved next time:

▶ "I'm glad I tried using a blindfold, but I don't think I'll do that again."
▶ "I enjoyed trying bondage, but my wrists were bound too tight. Next time let's try a different position, or something looser."
▶ "I know orgasms aren't a sure thing for my body, but next time I'd like to spend more focused time trying to get there."

If you're up for it, the next step is to make a plan for next time that includes your modifications:

▶ "How about next weekend we try tying you up?"
▶ "Let's do the same thing again, but a little slower, and with more warm-up."
▶ "Next time I'd love to play with more dirty talk, and hear what's hot for you while we're touching."

With this system, you can keep modifying the things you're trying until you're having the experience you'd like to have. And while I don't think perfection is a useful concept when it comes to sex, practice does make improvement!

SHARING SECRETS AND SEXUAL HISTORIES

Like we talked about early on, sharing secrets is one of the ways we build intimacy. And it doesn't need to be a secret in the literal sense. Anything that feels a little vulnerable or scary to share will do. For many folks, sharing anything about sexual fantasies or our sexual histories fits that bill.

I remember in high school, and maybe even college, a popular "truth or dare" question was to ask how many people someone had kissed or had sex with. As adults, many of us don't keep count. We're not collecting notches on our belts or our bed frames. But many of us do have highlights from our sexual histories that we like to share. A highlight might be an encounter that felt especially good, an exciting new thing that we tried, or a novel experience that makes for a great story.

Do you share these stories with your current partner(s)? Or do you prefer to treat each relationship like a blank slate? For me, at a minimum, I share and ask enough information to cover the sexual safety bases, but stories don't always go beyond that.

Most of us enjoy sharing our stories. Our experiences are a huge part of what makes us who we are, and telling someone else about these defining moments helps us feel seen. We can also learn a lot about another person by hearing their stories. Not only for the facts and the details they share, but by knowing what feels important or meaningful to them.

Sharing our sexual histories, in particular, can feel risky. Most people fear being judged—whether for how much experience they've had, or how little. Sexual experience is a double-edged sword in our culture. People get shamed for too much and too little. But there's no such thing as a right number of partners to have had. Some folks like exploring with a lot of people and others don't. It's all okay, as long as you're being true to yourself and what feels right to you.

If you'd like to try a secret-sharing/trust-building exercise with your partner, sharing details of your sexual history can be a good topic to play with. It can feel a little taboo and risky while also being a way to exchange useful information.

If you're going to give this a try, you need to be sure you can hear the information in a nonjudgmental way. You can't agree to the exchange and then shame your partner, or use the information they give you against them. So if you know you have biases or hang-ups you're still working through, this might not be the exercise for you.

If, however, you enjoy hearing about your partner's adventures, this could be a good fit. It can also be a good exercise to try if you're thinking about having a threesome, or group sex, or swinging with another couple— any situation where you think jealousy could be an issue. This way, you're able to test your reactions to hearing about your partner being with other people while it's in the past, and before anyone else's feelings are on the line in the here and now.

If you you've decided to go for it, choose the parameters. What stories do you want to share? A complete sexual history might be too much for one conversation. And the point isn't to come clean about everything you've ever done, it's to share stories you're excited about and that give your partner(s) information about who you are.

With that in mind, aim for qualitative rather than quantitative questions. Here are some conversation starters:

> Talk about your first kiss or the first time you had sex. Who was it with? How did you feel about it? What were the highlights?

> Talk about one of your favorite sexual encounters. This isn't about comparison! Just talk about what happened, who it was with, and what was hot about it.

> Talk about someone you had a crush on—someone in your real life or a character/celebrity.

> Talk about a sexual fantasy you have that you've never tried. Why is it sexy to you?

These are just a few ideas to get you started—feel free to modify them or make up your own. The point of the exercise is to share something about yourself and learn more about your partner.

DIRTY TALK

Dirty talk comes up again and again as a way to spice up long-distance relationships, communicate during sex, and incorporate difficult fantasies. But how do you actually do it? For people who are terrified of having the safer-sex talk, busting out with dialogue that sounds like it came from porn might seem downright ridiculous.

But dirty talk doesn't need to be done in a voice other than your own. It doesn't need to come from role play, a character, or anything that feels fake or put on. You can use your normal speaking voice, or a whisper, whatever feels most comfortable to you.

So what do you actually say? My personal favorite is to ask questions. This helps sneak in some extra check-ins, and it also shares the weight of keeping the talk going with the other person or people involved. I'll ask questions like, "Do you like that?" and "Do you want some more?" These questions can double (or triple?) as dirty talk, pleasure/consent check-ins, and even a bit of a playful tease, depending on how you say it. For me, this fits with my personality and my sexual persona. You'll need to try a few things to see what feels like a good fit for you.

When Dan Savage is giving advice about dirty talk, he suggests the following formula:

1) Say what you're going to do
2) Say what you're doing
3) Say what you did

That might sound incredibly simple, but it works. Most people are so unused to hearing sex words said out loud that even the most basic talk about what's going on can feel taboo and sexy. If you combine the "say what you're going to do" with the question asking from above, it also becomes an even more clear check-in and gives the person a chance to say no or to ask for something else instead.

So what would that look like in practice? Here's one example of following the above script:

1) "I'm going to give you the best massage you've ever had. Your skin is going to feel so good under my fingers, all slippery with the massage oil. I can just see how tense your muscles are and how badly you need this. Does that sound good? Do you want a massage? Say please."

2) "I knew it, your skin feels so good sliding under my hands. I love digging my fingers into your muscles and hearing you moan as I touch you. Does this feel good? Do you want me to squeeze harder? I can feel all your tense spots just melting under my fingers."

3) "I just loved giving you a massage. Thank you for letting me do that. Was it fun for you, too? Could I give you a massage again sometime?"

Complimenting your partner is usually a safe bet, as long as you're minding any requests they've made about ways you describe their body. You can also use compliments as a way to reassure people about things they might be self-conscious about—and during sex, that can be most things. But generally people like to hear they look good naked and that their bodies smell and taste good.

You can also simply describe what you're feeling at that moment, or talk about what things you're doing that feel good. If you're sticking to what's actually happening, you don't need to rack your brain for outrageous fantasies to describe—all the material you need is right in front of you. Here are some examples:

- ▸ "Your skin feels amazing."
- ▸ "I love how your breath/mouth/hands feel on my body."
- ▸ "It feels amazing to be so close to you."
- ▸ "I'm so turned on."
- ▸ "I love watching your fingers clench the sheets."
- ▸ "I love touching you."

- ▸ "I love hearing the sounds you make."
- ▸ "You smell/taste so good."
- ▸ "Your body feels incredible under my hands."
- ▸ "That's so good, please don't stop."
- ▸ "I love that—please do it harder."

You'll notice that in the last couple of examples, I sneaked in ways you can make requests while couching them in compliments/dirty talk so that they fit with the flow of what's going on. It's not that tricky once you get the hang of it. You just need to give yourself permission to feel a little silly while you're getting used to it.

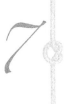

Tools and Hands-On Exercises

EXERCISE—ASK FOR EVERYTHING

WHEN YOU AREN'T IN THE HABIT OF ASKING FOR what you want, it can be a daunting prospect. But there are lots of ways to start building your asking muscles, and many of them can be a lot of fun! One of my favorite exercises to suggest to clients is one where they have to ask for every little thing they want.

You'll want to share with your partner that this is what you're doing, and it's also great if you can take turns being the asker and the receiver. It's also helpful to start with things that feel low stakes. Maybe sitting next to each other on the couch or on the floor. Start by asking to hold hands, or maybe for a hand massage. You can ask for a shoulder massage or to have your neck kissed.

Step by step, keep asking for the things you want next, with the understanding that nothing at all will happen that you don't ask for. Eventually maybe you'll feel comfortable with clothes coming off, and with more sexually charged touch. Hopefully, if you take your time getting to genital touch, you'll feel comfortable asking for the specific kinds of touch that you like in that area, too.

As you're doing this, you also want to build the habit of thanking your partner for feedback. We can be so worried that asking for something will hurt our partner's feelings that it can be great to have the reinforcement that they're grateful for the information. You'll have to find the language that's comfortable for you, but thanking someone for feedback is a powerful tool and one that will encourage getting more feedback in the future.

EXERCISE—GIVE FEEDBACK

Very similar to the ask-for-everything exercise, this exercise is for getting you used to giving feedback on what's happening. Again, you want to make it clear that this is what you're going to be doing. And again, doing it with something low stakes, like a massage, is a great way to practice before moving to something sexual.

The basic pattern here is to first say what you'd like: "Could I please have a back rub?" Then when your partner is touching you, make a request for some kind of adjustment—harder, softer, etc.

When the adjustment is made, one or both people can say thank you. It can be nice to take turns. The idea is to reinforce that making requests is a good thing, not an imposition. Our partners are generally thrilled to know exactly what we'd like. It takes the pressure off them to guess or to try to read our minds. People usually want to do things that make us feel good. So letting them know what that is helps everyone out.

Imagine something like this:

David is sitting at the kitchen table, and Paul stands behind him. David asks, "Would you please rub my shoulders?"

Paul responds, "I'd love to, thanks for asking me," and begins to squeeze.

"Would you use a little more pressure?" David asks, and Paul does, digging his hands deeper into the muscles and saying, "Thank you for telling me what you want."

I keep using massage as an example, and I encourage you to do so as well, because so many of the same terms and requests apply. Harder and softer, left and right, etc. Not only that, but it's an activity we do to give and receive pleasure, so even when there are no sexual components, it can mean we're in a similar mind-set, which can make it easier to transfer these skills into our bedrooms and our sex lives.

SHOW, DON'T TELL

If you've ever been in a writing class or read a book about writing techniques, you've heard the phrase "show, don't tell." In writing, this means being more descriptive. You don't say, "It was a cold day." You say, "Nate stepped outside and could see his breath form a fog as it left his mouth. His nose and fingers prickled, and he hurried to tuck his scarf around his neck and pull his gloves out of his pockets."

You get the idea. One is simply more interesting. It pulls you into the world. It makes you feel what the character is feeling. And we tend to believe things we experience, more than things we're told, even if we're experiencing them through descriptive language on a page.

Show, don't tell, is even more valuable when it comes to sex and bodies. In this case I'm using it as an easy way to remember the concept, because of course I want you to tell, also. This book is largely about using your words. Even so, words can't fully replace showing a concrete example of what we mean.

When you're getting to know someone's body for the first time, you have the tools you've learned with other partners—if you've had other partners. You have everything you've learned about sex from movies, porn, books, talking to friends, and exploring with your own body. But everyone is different, and there's always nuance to how someone likes to be touched. The very best way to learn how someone likes to be touched is to watch them touch themselves.

This can be scary for a lot of people. Being watched can make us feel more vulnerable, or more self-conscious, than having sex. When we're mutually engaged in a sexual activity, there are distractions. But when someone watches us touch ourselves, all of their attention is on us. The lights are up enough to see, and there are no distractions.

It's understandable if that feels like too much for you at first. I think it's worth working up to, if you can, both because it is a valuable tool and because when something feels vulnerable and scary, going through it with a partner helps us build intimacy.

Here are some ways to help you have a comfortable experience when masturbating in front of a partner for the first time.

Set aside time specifically for this, so there won't be distractions. Pick a time that won't feel rushed, and when you're well rested, well fed, and in a good mood. Talk about what the parameters will be. Decide if it's best just to touch yourself while your partner watches quietly, or if you'd feel better talking through it. Do you want to narrate what you're doing? Do you want your partner to ask questions? Think about what will make you feel most comfortable, and don't forget that you can always change your mind.

Set up the room in a way that feels sexy and comfortable. Think about the lighting, maybe using candles or something else that casts a warm glow. Set the temperature to something that will feel comfortable on bare skin. Arrange everything you'll need within easy reach—lube, sex toys, a towel, whatever is part of your normal process. It will be helpful to not have to stop and look for things once you get started.

Decide what positions will be most comfortable. It can help to be in the same position you'd usually be in when touching yourself. So you'll need to find the best way for your partner to watch with a good view, but without getting in the way or being too close for comfort.

Also decide whether you want to fool around together at all as foreplay, or if you'd like to keep this encounter purely instructive. It can also be a good idea to negotiate what will happen afterward. Your partner might be turned on by watching you, so will you two want to play together after the demonstration, or will they take a turn demonstrating what they like next?

Considering and negotiating all of these details in advance is your best chance for things to move smoothly and to avoid any surprises or hurt feelings in the moment.

When it comes to the actual touch, take your time.

Remember that it's incredibly sexy and intimate to share in this way. So don't feel like you need to rush or like your partner will be bored or impatient. If you can, try to enjoy the process of being watched. Or if it's easier for you, close your eyes or wear a blindfold so you can forget your audience. Touch yourself the way you would when you're alone. Let your partner see how you use your hands, what parts of your body enjoy touch, and what kinds of touches you use. People think some of this is obvious, but as we've already demonstrated, nothing is obvious when it comes to bodies and sex. You may never have thought of some of the details that go into what kind of touch you like.

If you have a clit, do you usually touch the right side, the left side, or both? Or do you focus on other kinds of sensations—maybe all-over grinding or focusing on the labia or on penetration. Maybe you don't even use your hands—maybe you focus on stimulation with toys.

If you have a penis, how do you usually hold it? Do you use one hand or two? Do you use lube or enjoy some friction? What speed do you like to be stroked?

If you're trans or genderqueer, it can be even more important to talk about and show what you like, because there can be so much variation.

For many of us, masturbation is so second nature that we don't really think about what we do. And that's part of why it can be hard to tell someone else what we like, because we haven't really thought about it. So going through this process is also a chance for you to think about what you're doing and figure out how you'd put words to the things you enjoy. Even if you're not talking during the process, think about things like speed and pressure so that the next time your partner is touching you, you'll have an idea of what to ask for.

LEARN SOMETHING NEW TOGETHER

When it comes to sex, we feel like we're supposed to know it all already. It can be hard to admit there's something we need to learn, or need to work on, because our ego takes a beating. As we've established, *the perfect is the enemy of the good.*

But there's a trick to getting around that feeling. By trying something that our ego isn't invested in, something that we have no reason to know how to do, we can give ourselves permission to be a beginner.

Various kinks can be especially useful for this, because most of us didn't learn rope bondage, flogging, or fire cupping in high school or college. We can approach these activities (and many others) with wide eyes and an open mind.

When you've found something new that you'd like to learn, there can be great value to learning a new skill with your partner. Even if it's not sexy or kinky, learning something new (chess, scuba diving, rock climbing, a new language) helps stimulate parts of our brain, and it becomes a shared project. Not only are shared hobbies and activities a great way to maintain ongoing connection, but studies have shown that experiencing novelty helps keep a relationship alive. Even something as simple as trying a new restaurant together can go a long way.

So learning a new sex or kink skill together does double duty. One of my favorite skills to teach couples is rope bondage. There are a few reasons for this. First, it fits the bill for novelty and also for something we don't feel like we should know already. Secondly, rope gives you a reason to be up close and personal with someone, and it gives you a road map for how to touch someone's body, so it can be perfect for people who are trying to build or rebuild intimacy.

Rope can also be done over clothes, and there doesn't need to be any overtly sexual contact, so it can feel safer for people who are coming back from any difficult feelings around sex or nudity.

When you choose something that's new to both of you, you're on the same page and aren't in the position of comparing your skill or competency. And as you learn, it becomes not only something you can enjoy together, but also something you can take pride in the process of learning.

LAUGHTER AND PLAYFULNESS

Sex can be silly. Bodies can do silly things. It can be incredibly helpful to keep a lighthearted mind-set and be ready to accept anything that your body or your partner's body throws at you. Bodies make noises, and they make messes. And they don't always perform exactly the way you'd like them to. All of these possibilities are things you're best off being ready for, so that a normal bodily response doesn't derail a whole sexual experience or lead to embarrassment or shame.

It can help to be prepared to laugh in the bedroom. I think taking a lighthearted approach to sex and kink play can be a great way to take some of the pressure off. We get so serious about sex and kink, and that pressure can make it harder to try new things.

To set a light tone and encourage laughter, try playing games in the bedroom. Did you know they make Twister bedsheets? Those could provide hours of silly fun. Your local sex shop also probably carries games you can try. From card games to dice games, sometimes found in the party sections, these games can help you loosen up and try new things. Keep in mind some of them are probably terrible, but it's okay to take the parts you like and ignore the rest.

Want to play some games without going shopping? There are a lot of ways you can get playful in the bedroom without any props, or with things you probably have around the house.

Roll the dice

Have you got some dice? Assign a meaning for each number on the die—maybe one dot is kissing, two dots is massage, etc. Assign something for each number and also decide how long each activity will last. (If you want to get more advanced, you can use the other die to roll for time.) This game can have you kissing for two minutes, rubbing feet for five minutes, and then brushing someone's hair for three minutes. You can assign activities that are as tame or as wild as you want, as long as everyone agrees to them. Part of the fun can be moving from something like hair brushing to something like oral sex, and then back to something like scratching your partner's back. This can disrupt the idea that sex play only progresses in one direction, toward genital stimulation and orgasm. You could do the same thing with a deck of cards, too, using the different suits or numbers for the different activities.

Sensational

This is a game that can help you focus on sensation using just things you've got around your house. You can take turns collecting items while making sure your partner doesn't see what you've grabbed. Think feathers, fur, flowers, maybe ice cubes and something you can warm up. Kitchen implements, hairbrushes . . . anything that's body safe and has a unique feel. Then you and your partner take turns being blindfolded and having the mystery objects slid along your skin. Can you identify what they are? Feel free to get playfully competitive about it and assign a reward for whichever one of you is able to identify more of the items.

Playful role play

You might be used to role play as part of kink, or as part of your current sexual repertoire. Maybe professor/student or doctor/nurse. But for this game, you want to pick something silly. Something where it might be difficult to keep a straight face, or to think of a plot line that makes any sense. Dog and dogcatcher, maybe? Car and car mechanic? The point of this one is to get used to being silly, and laughing, and having it be okay that not everything is supersexy.

NONVERBAL COMMUNICATION

When I was working on my sociology degree in college, nonverbal communication was one of my specialties. The classes on this topic were taught by my mentor and favorite teacher, and I even helped produce several documentaries on the topic that were used in classroom settings.

Just like verbal language, nonverbal language is culturally specific. You can't make assumptions with someone's nonverbal cues any more than you can make assumptions on other topics. In fact, some gestures have fundamentally opposite meanings in different cultures. For example, the hand gesture that folks in America consider the peace sign is the symbol for "up yours" in England.

While nonverbal communication is a huge part of any sexual encounter, it's also an area that is very prone to going wrong. All too often people assume someone wanted something, or was enjoying something, based on their interpretation of nonverbal cues.

Nonverbal cues are never a substitute for verbal negotiation and check-ins. This section talks about ways to get to know someone's nonverbal cues better, but it assumes you're doing these things within the context of an existing, already negotiated, sexual relationship.

Sometimes a nonverbal cue is simply an indication that it's time for a verbal check-in. If someone's face is all scrunched up, that could indicate concentration, pain, or pleasure. It's safest to ask someone how they're feeling any time you're not sure.

Some cues you'll learn over time with a partner, and others you can ask about right away. It can be a good conversation to have before you have sex with someone— you can ask about their reactions and responses. Personally, I like to warn people that laughter is my response to just about everything, from pleasure to pain, before they get their feelings hurt or are lost in confusion.

I've had partners warn me about everything from shuddering to convulsing to whimpering so I'd know what to expect when they were experiencing pleasure. For some people, even crying is a good sign. But it's important to know that in advance, as well as what your partner would like you to do when they have any of these responses.

Although there are no sure things, you can learn to

look out for what are usually happy sounds and noises. Moans and gasps and even purring. Maybe the first time you hear a new sound, you ask, "Is that a good thing?" And then based on the answer, you can use that response to let you know when you're on the right track.

Another thing that is often, though not always, a good sign is when someone's body language opens up, giving you more access to various parts of their body. You can also look for things like swelling, flushing, and even lubrication. There are no surefire signs of arousal, so there's no way to get around asking, but once you learn someone's cues, you can look out for them in the future.

Want to play with nonverbal cues in a tangible way? I learned an exercise during my intimacy-educator training that you can try for yourself. When we did it, one student would lie on a massage table with two or three people around them. The person lying down would keep their arms at their sides if they only wanted PG-13 areas of their bodies to be touched, and would raise their arms above their heads if everywhere was fair game. They were also encouraged to change back and forth a few times, to escalate and deescalate the level of touch being given.

You can decide what kind of touch makes the most sense for you. When we did the exercise in my training, we used open-handed caressing, or touching with just the tips of our fingers. As the exercise progresses, the person being touched learns that they can control what's happening to them, that they have agency over their experience. The person doing the touching has a chance to practice watching for nonverbal cues. And both people get experience with touch being something that can both escalate or deescalate during an encounter.

You can try this at home either by using the movement of your arms as the cue or with the nonverbal signal of your choice. It can be a good tool for having nonverbal ways to slow down or speed up what's happening, for people who find talking during sex a challenge.

SLOW DOWN

Whatever you're doing, try doing it slower.

In my classes I run people though an exercise where I ask students to stroke their own arm at a pace they consider to be sensual. Then I tell them to do the same thing at half the speed and ask what differences they notice.

While everyone is different, and slower isn't always better, it's a valuable exercise to try, because you're able to experience more sensations. The skin being touched can feel things more acutely, and the hand or fingers doing the touching can also focus on sensation more. Another fun result of this experiment is that the skin that's about to be touched can experience anticipation, which for many people is part of the fun.

Going slowly also gives the person being touched time to process what's happening, and it gives them more time to speak up if they want a change. Many people have had countless experiences of things going a lot faster than they'd like, and it's not unusual to be on guard in a sexual encounter for the moment something will go too fast or become uncomfortable.

If you can move at a slow pace, it lets the other person relax and savor the experience, knowing that nothing will happen faster than they have a chance to react.

And although a quickie is fun now and then, there's a great deal of pleasure to be accessed when you take more time for the arousal process. Although explicit research into sexual functioning is lacking, there's evidence that it can take the clitoral complex as much as thirty to forty minutes to be fully engorged. And that level of arousal is what it takes for some people to enjoy penetration. While this is just one example, a variety of bodies need more time to become relaxed and aroused in order to experience the full range of pleasure they are capable of.

If nothing else, it's a lot safer to go too slow than too fast. The worst that can happen is that your partner will urge you to do more, and that's a great position to be in.

Need some help slowing things down? Try setting a timer and see what it feels like to focus on only kissing, or only touching, for a set period of time. For this exercise avoid genital contact. Just focus on the other ways you can explore each other's bodies. You can start by just doing this for five minutes, and each time you play, you can add three to five minutes to the clock. You can make it a game to see how long you can play with just kissing and touching before you're too eager to wait for other things.

PRACTICE WITH A PARTY

If you're game to make out with your friends, throwing a party can be a great way to practice some of your communication and negotiation skills! At the parties I cohost and attend, we've adapted our own consent-focused version of spin the bottle, and I think it's a fabulous tool for anyone to use. Here's how it goes: you spin the bottle the way you're used to, and when it lands on someone, the spinner makes a proposal. Then the spinnee can accept the proposal or make a counteroffer.

This version of the game eliminates the coercion and peer pressure from the original and gives you an opportunity to practice the skills of asking for what you want, and for negotiating.

Here's an example of how it works at parties:

Mitch spins the bottle, and it lands on Fiona. Mitch asks, "Would you like a kiss on the mouth?"

Fiona thinks about it and answers, "Actually, I'd prefer a kiss on the cheek," and Mitch leans forward to oblige. Now it's Fiona's turn to spin. The bottle lands on Jasmine, and Fiona asks, "Would you like to bend over and get three spanks on your ass?"

Jasmine giggles and answers, "Yes, please!" and bends over to receive her spankings.

With each round of the game, people get more comfortable making requests, and having it be reinforced that making a counterrequest is not only okay, it's encouraged.

If you don't want to do it with a group of people, you can even do it with one other person, just taking turns making requests and then accepting those requests or making a counteroffer.

If you do like the party idea, there are a few other ways you can start getting a little sexier with your circle of friends. It doesn't mean you have to launch into all-out orgies, but many people find that it's valuable to start being more open with their friends and peers around topics of sex and sexuality.

When you're ready to get started, make sure you start

with something easy. Hosting a movie night with a sexy film and a chance to talk about it afterward can be a great icebreaker. Maybe you have friends who are interested in kink? Get together and watch *Secretary,* and then share your feedback.

Not only is this a fun way to spend an evening, but it can make talking about sex and sexuality with your friends easier, which is valuable when you want someone to talk to about your own sex life and relationships.

Another way to have a sexy party is to invite people over for erotica reading. Encourage everyone to bring something to share, whether it's a section of a favorite book or something they found online. Then after mingling and snacks, people take turns getting up in front of the group and reading their story aloud. This works best with stories that don't take longer than five minutes to read, otherwise you might start to lose people's attention, and it's a long time for one person to be on the spot.

After everyone has gotten a chance to share, the group can talk about their favorites as well as the stories they had strong reactions to. It can be incredibly interesting to see a room full of people all having different responses to the same content, and with a few ground rules about not being judgmental, it can also be a great way to practice talking about the kind of things that turn us on and turn us off.

For people who want to get this energy going but don't want to host, you can also find sex-positive events in your town that you can attend with friends. From storytelling shows to burlesque, many areas have a wide range of events to choose from. You can attend the event with your friends and then go out for drinks afterward to share your reactions and feelings.

Trying any or all of these things is a great way to get more comfortable talking about sex, and sexy topics, and it can foster a great deal of openness among your friends. Without even knowing it, you could be helping people release shame or fear they've been holding onto about sex and sexuality for their whole lives!

IMPROVISATION

Part of the resistance to communicating about sex, and asking for what you want, is that people think that means you can never improvise. That's certainly not what I'm suggesting. Part of why we negotiate our yeses and noes is so that we can improvise within those bounds, without checking in every time we move our hand an inch. You can practice playing with this, too. Like with so many things, using massage can be a great way to start.

Think about setting the parameters for a massage: you talk about what parts of your body you'd like to have as the focus, which ones are off-limits, and what kind of pressure you'd like. From there, the massage therapist will probably check in once or twice about the pressure they're using, but the massage will mostly pass in silence.

You can try this in your own play by setting up smaller scenarios and then improvising within them. You can use massage as the activity to play with, or any kind of sensual touch. Here's an example of how that could go:

You agree to a massage anywhere on the body that isn't covered by undergarments. You want moderate pressure and a focus on shoulders and neck. Then, the person doing the touching has a wide range of areas at their disposal, as well as knowing what boundaries they're working within.

However you decide to play, just remember that the

suggestions in these exercises aren't meant to restrain creativity, but to give you more tools to express it safely.

Want to borrow an activity used in theatrical improvisation? There's a well-known game called "yes, and." The idea is that the performers build a scene by agreeing to whatever the previous performer has said (that's the "yes" part) and then adding their own statement, (that's the "and"). Using these tools, the performers will build absurd stories and scenarios.

If you're trying this in the bedroom, make sure your boundaries are clear in advance so both people know what to ask for. (And no matter what the title implies, you can always say no.) Then, like a cousin to the "ask for everything" exercise, you take turns building a sexual scenario together. It might go something like this:

"Would you kiss me on the neck?"

"Yes, and may I stroke your hair?"

"Yes, and may I touch your chest?"

"Yes, and may I remove your shirt?"

You can take this as far as both people want, depending on what boundaries were established about playing the game. It's okay if it feels silly—in fact, I encourage giggles and laughter.

AROUSAL TRACKING

When I ask people what turns them on, they often don't have an answer. Most people haven't really thought about it before. And I don't just mean the sexual fantasies we've already worked through. I also mean the smaller, daily things like putting on an outfit that makes you feel confident or sexy, or something that has fabric that feels good against your skin. Maybe it's taking a bath or a shower, or feeling fresh air or sunshine on your skin.

If you go through your day thinking about your arousal states, you'll learn a lot about how your body functions. It's probably no surprise that when you're tired, stressed, or sore, you don't feel very sexy. And when you're relaxed, well rested, and feel good in your skin, you're more willing to engage with other people. When you start to learn your turn-ons and turnoffs, it gets easier to plan to be in a sexy space when you want to be.

You can do this exercise by carrying a little notebook or using your phone to track how you're feeling. You just need one column for what's going on and another for how aroused or sexy you're feeling on a scale of one to ten. Aroused doesn't have to mean that you're interested in sex or an orgasm right at that moment. It can just be a state of being in your body, how you feel in your skin. Maybe a mood that would make you want to experience something sensual, either alone or with a partner.

Here are some times of day or scenarios you could track:

> - When you first wake up, the feeling of your sheets against your body.
> - When you're in the shower, feeling the water on your skin.
> - When you get dressed in the morning.
> - Drinking a cup of coffee.
> - Walking out the front door and feeling the air on your face.
> - Standing in the sunshine.
> - Meeting a deadline or feeling productive at work.

> ▸ Enjoying a favorite meal.
> ▸ Working out.
> ▸ Putting on your pajamas and snuggling up on the couch.
> ▸ Sliding into bed at night.

These suggestions are just a way to get you started thinking about all of your experiences throughout the day. You can list whatever items happen to come up for you. And although most of my suggestions are positive experiences, it's also valuable to track the things that are turnoffs—maybe getting stuck in traffic or getting in a fight. Because your turnoffs are just as valuable to know about when you want to track your overall mood.

Another way you can track your arousal is against factors like stress or energy. Rather than tracking specific things that are happening, you can summarize any given moment based on a few data points. Maybe during the week you have a chart that looks like this:

Energy: 8   Stress: 5   Arousal: 6

Tracking in this way, you can have proof whether getting more sleep, or being less stressed, affects your eagerness for intimacy or sex. And based on this information, you can try to set yourself up for the best chance of a good time when you schedule dates or special events.

Sometimes even with all of this information, getting in the mood is still a big project. If, for example, you realize you need to reduce stress to feel like having sex, that's easier said than done. But it's still helpful to know what you're working toward to be able to take steps in that direction.

WHAT MAKES YOU FEEL SEXY?

Once you've done the arousal tracking, you'll start to have an idea how your mood shifts throughout the day and what affects it. But our deliberate choices make a difference, too. There are things we can ask for and scenarios we can set up that will increase our chances of feeling in the mood.

Maybe it sounds cliché to dim the lights and burn candles, but it's a cliché because it works for a lot of people. Flattering lighting makes people feel more comfortable naked. And there's no reason not to set up your space in the ways that feel ideal to you. From light to music to fragrance, play with different things until you find what works for you.

Choosing outfits you feel good in can also help. Most of us have something that makes us feel our best, so pay attention when you figure out what that is, and use it to your advantage when you need some extra help. If you're not yet sure what your power outfits are (or maybe your power lingerie or underwear), set some time aside to play dress up in your own closet. Sometimes we haven't viewed our clothes as more than utilitarian, and shifting our focus can unearth gems we didn't know were there.

Is there a kind of compliment you especially enjoy from your partner? Or a way that they touch you that makes you feel wanted? If you don't know the answer, try to look out for this over time. Journaling or tracking your responses in a notebook can be useful for this. But even making mental notes can work, too.

When your partner greets you on date night with a tender hug and a kiss on the cheek, how do you feel? When they greet you with a tight squeeze and a passionate kiss, how do you feel?

There are no right or wrong answers here, only a way to begin noticing how we read nonverbal communication and physical cues. As with most things, our partners are usually grateful when we tell them what makes us feel loved and wanted, so share this information when you figure it out.

HOW TO MAKE UNREALISTIC FANTASIES, OR SOMETHING ONLY ONE PERSON WANTS, HAPPEN

In the "What Do You Want" section, we went through a lot of ways to get at the core of what's sexy to you, sometimes in surprising ways. But sometimes we come upon fantasies that are so logistically challenging, physically dangerous, or ethically dubious that engaging in them in any meaningful way simply isn't possible.

All hope is not lost! I'm sure you've heard it said that the brain is the biggest sex organ, and in this case that's really helpful.

One of my favorite ways to access fantasies that you can't act out in your real life is through written erotica. One of the powerful things about reading your smut (versus watching porn) is that you can fill in a lot of the blanks yourself. You imagine the characters in a way that's appealing to you, and it's harder to get distracted by the indifferent cat that walks into the shot—seemingly a mainstay of amateur porn.

With erotica, anything is possible. From unicorns to centaurs to anything else you can imagine, it's all available on the page. If you can't find what you're looking for already in print, there are even services that will custom write erotica for you, in line with whatever fetishes or kinks you specify.

Animated or illustrated smut is another way to go. There are many erotic comics to choose from, and once again fantastical creatures (and other hard-to-manage scenarios) can easily take place.

Whatever form of erotic content you choose, from live-action porn to written erotica, you can also decide whether you want to enjoy it alone or include your partner. This can lead to valuable conversations about each person's turn-ons and interests.

If your partner is game, working fantasies into dirty talk is another great way to explore your turn-ons without acting them out. Whether you decide to role-play the scenarios of your dreams or simply spin erotic stories out loud, this can come surprisingly close to the real thing.

In my first sexual relationship, this fantasy building was a mainstay of our sex life. My partner had a variety of kinks and we'd incorporate them this way—I'd spin elaborate stories while I used my hands on him. Add a blindfold and the imagination does the rest of the work for you.

Not only are these methods useful for accessing fantasies that can't be enacted in real life, these methods can also be a way to incorporate fantasies that only one person is into.

Sure, there are some things we simply want no part of,

and that's fine. But sometimes there are things we don't physically want to do but don't mind talking about or reading about. When that's the case, using porn, erotica, or dirty talk can be a great way for someone to get their kinky fantasies and needs met without their partner doing anything they aren't comfortable with.

And sometimes even that level of involvement is too much. Sometimes our partners are into something that we simply don't want to engage in, in any way. When that's the case, there's a larger conversation to be had about how to manage that. Asking someone to not fully express their sexuality isn't fair, but there are other ways it can work that don't involve the uninterested party.

The easiest solution is to find a way for someone to get their fantasies met on their own. Maybe through porn or erotica they watch on their own, or though things they incorporate into their masturbation routine. Beyond that comes a discussion of relationship boundaries. If it's already an open relationship, that can make it easy for someone to get different needs met with different people. But if you're not interested in being fully open, there may be some room for compromise. What about someone being involved with another person who only engages in the kink or fetish with them, but doesn't have sex or a relationship?

In the kink scenes of most cities, you'll find people who go to get certain experiences without necessarily dating the people they play with. There's a conversation to be had there, as well, to make sure that's what the other person is game for. But sometimes it's the perfect alignment of kinks and boundaries.

If that's still farther than you want to go, there's also the option of hiring a professional. You can find people who work in phone sex or cam work who are well versed in a variety of different kinks and fetishes, and sometimes that's the perfect compromise. On the one hand, it's a real person to engage in the fantasies with, and on the other they're still kept at a distance, being on the phone or online rather than physically with you.

Whatever route you choose to go, make sure the conversation is had with empathy and care, not to shame people who have interests different from yours.

INTRODUCING SEX TOYS

As a sex educator, my house is overflowing with sex toys. It becomes a storage problem. I've even got an over-the-door shoe holder repurposed to hold vibrators and dildos. So from my happy sex-toy bubble, sometimes it's hard to remember that only twenty five to fifty percent of people have tried using sex toys, depending on which study you want to believe.

It's a shame, because sex toys are amazing tools. Like any other tool, they're specially made to get a particular job done. There are vibrators for internal or external use, dildos, butt plugs, masturbation sleeves, and more. In fact, there are so many toys available that sometimes it's hard to know where to start.

First, why might you want to use sex toys? Sex toys can be a great tool to use alone to figure out all the ways your body can experience pleasure and might be able to reach orgasm. If you're interested in internal stimulation, like G-spot or prostate play, those areas can be hard to reach on our own bodies. But toys made for those exact purposes do a wonderful job and save you the carpal tunnel of trying to reach them with your fingers.

Some people need particular kinds of intense stimulation to get aroused or reach orgasm, whether that's just how they're built or they are influenced by medications, surgeries, or other body changes over time. In these cases, sometimes toys are the only way to get the kind of stimulation needed.

Whatever the reason, toys can bring a whole new dimension to solo or partnered sex and are well worth giving a try. But despite their utility, there's still a stigma about sex toys. There are pervasive beliefs that using toys somehow spoils you for partnered sex, or that only people who are disappointed in their partners want to use toys. None of these ideas hold water.

Not only do toys not ruin you for partnered play, but anything that helps get you in touch with the pleasure your body can experience actually helps enhance partnered play—with or without toys. And although self-reporting studies about sex are notoriously flawed, evidence suggests that couples who use sex toys together report higher satisfaction with their sex lives.

"A 2016 study conducted by Chapman University's David Frederick, PhD, found that women and men who reported feeling satisfied by their relationship and the sex that they had with their partners were more likely to report having used sex toys together—in addition to other activities, such as taking a shower together, trying new positions in bed, and scheduling a date night to have sex."[5]

---

5   Katherine Schreiber and Heather Hausenblas, PhD. "How Sex Toys Impact Relationships," *Psychology Today* (blog), May 27, 2017, https://www.psychologytoday.com/blog/the-truth-about-exercise-addiction/201705/how-sex-toys-impact-relationships.

Having toys in your toolbox means having even more options to choose from when you're deciding what kind of sex you want to have. And having more options increases your chances of finding something that works for everybody more often. Not only that, but toys can be a great option when one person is tired or wants a quickie, or when someone's body isn't doing exactly what they'd like it to. Toys give you a great deal more flexibility about the ways you can interact.

So how do you broach the subject with your partner? If you don't have toys already, going shopping together can make for a fun and sexy date, and picking something out together can sometimes help it feel like more of a couple's toy.

If you have a toy already that you'd like to introduce into your partnered play, it doesn't have to be a big deal. You can use any of the techniques we've already discussed for bringing up things you'd like to try. People expect their partners to be threatened by toys, but you can head that off before it happens by reminding your partner you enjoy the sex you're having already and would just like to play with trying something new.

Another way to make toys feel less threatening is to let your partner drive them, at least at first. Whether it's holding the vibrator, or the stroker, or the plug, you can find ways for your partner to use the toy as an extension of themselves.

There are also toys that are specifically made to be couples' toys, but in my experience those usually aren't the best ones. They often have tricky ways they're meant to attach to one person's body or the other, and they tend to have a higher learning curve to make them successful.

The best bet is to stick with something simple at first, and as you develop more of an idea of what you and your partner enjoy, you can use that information to add to your bag of tricks.

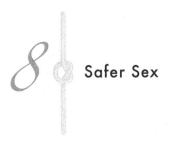

8   Safer Sex

WHY TALK ABOUT SAFETY?

ONE OF THE CONVERSATIONS PEOPLE SEEM TO dread the most is about safer sex and STI status. In fact, when I teach my Modern Dating class, people tell me that in their experience, people aren't having these talks at all. That's distressing for many reasons. For one, without talking about risk, it's much harder to keep yourself safe. And if you feel like you can't talk about safety and sexually transmitted infections with a partner, how are you going to talk about pleasure and what kind of touch you like? Skipping this conversation sets a bad precedent.

I find that in the kink and open relationship communities, people have gotten more used to this kind of communication and negotiation. In part I think this is because when people are used to engaging in higher-risk behaviors like kink, or trickier situations like juggling multiple partners, talking about it is more common. I think it's also because people tend to put more effort into protecting others than themselves. So when the health of a partner is at stake, people are more on top of safety.

Having these conversations up front also sets the tone for honesty and transparency. One study showed that people who thought they were in monogamous relationships actually had a higher rate of STIs than people in open relationships. That's because people who were cheating weren't having safety talks with the people they were cheating with, often weren't using barriers, and certainly weren't talking to their spouses about these activities.[6]

Talking about safety is essential for your sexual wellbeing. The next two sections will show you how to figure out your personal risk tolerance and how to have this conversation with your partners.

RISK TOLERANCE

If you've ever done retirement planning or filled out 401(k) paperwork at your job, you've probably done a risk-tolerance worksheet. The idea is simple: they ask you a series of questions to determine how you'll react to various changes in the market. This information helps financial planners decide how aggressively to invest your money. If you have a high risk tolerance, they invest aggressively, aiming for long-term growth but knowing it might be a rocky ride. If you have low risk tolerance, they make safer choices that won't make as much money but also won't lose value.

You can use a similar process to conceptualize your risk tolerance when it comes to sexual safety and STI risk.

---

6   Justin J. Lehmiller, "A Comparison of Sexual Health History and Practices Among Monogamous and Consensually Nonmonogamous Sexual Partners," *The Journal of Sexual Medicine* 12, no. 10 (2015): 2022–2028. doi: 10.1111/jsm.12987.

Just like a financial planner might ask how you'd react if the market dips, ask yourself how you'd react if you were to contract an STI. Would it feel fairly straightforward to get tested, get treatment, and tell your partner(s)? Or would you feel like it's the end of the world?

Sit down and think about that for a minute. Imagine that you get a phone call from a partner saying they've tested positive for an STI, or that you've just gotten a positive test result yourself. How do you feel? When you think about making that call to someone else and telling them they need to get tested, how does that feel? Can you imagine having that conversation?

These are the kinds of things we need to be ready to talk about if we're going to be having sex with other people. There's no such thing as completely risk-free sex, even within a monogamous relationship. It's possible for things to have been dormant for years, or for something to crop up that someone was never tested for or can't be tested for.

Having sex with other people means accepting a certain amount of risk. It's one of the responsibilities we take on when we agree to have sex. And having sex responsibly means limiting our own risk and limiting the risks we're exposing other people to.

When you're assessing risk tolerance, one of the first things you need to figure out is how you define risk. Are you considering the likelihood of catching/transmitting STIs as your main risk factor, are you thinking about pregnancy, or do you have other concerns that enter into the equation?

Once you've determined your risk tolerance, you aren't done forever. Just like with financial risk tolerance, sexual risk tolerance changes over time. Maybe you feel one way when you're single and another when you've met someone you're really into. Maybe you feel one way when you're younger and another when you're older or planning a family. You'll need to return to this idea every so often and see what, if anything, has changed for you.

When you're having this conversation with your partner, you'll also have to figure out if your risk-tolerance levels are the same, or if you fall in different places. If they're different, you'll have to decide how to navigate that discrepancy as you're deciding on your safety protocols and your boundaries.

Part of accurately assessing your risk tolerance is being informed about what the actual risks are. You can read more information about STIs in the resources section through the links that are included. Keep in mind also that none of the risks are static—many of them are open to interpretation. With some STIs, the biggest issue is stigma, but with others, there can be serious health consequences. You'll need to gather all of that information so you can make an informed choice about how you want to mitigate your risks.

One of the best ways to get a clear picture of your sexual health is by visiting a sex-positive doctor you can talk to openly about your activities. You should also get a full STI testing panel so you can share that information with partners and potential partners, and so that you're already modeling that behavior when you ask for their test results.

When you're thinking about testing and frequency of

testing, it's important to consider the incubation period for various sexually transmitted infections. Some things can lay dormant for ninety days or more, so it can actually take two tests, ninety days apart, to be relatively sure someone has no infections. And even this isn't foolproof. Some infections or viruses can be dormant even longer or can be difficult to test for.

Knowing your personal risk tolerance—and the risk tolerance of your partner, if applicable—can help you decide how stringent your safer-sex protocols need to be. It's important to decide what makes you feel safe in advance so you're not making an impulsive decision when there's a person in front of you that you're eager to have sex with.

So here are some steps:

▸ Figure out your personal risk tolerance.
▸ Decide how often you want to get tested for STIs.
▸ Think about how often you want your partner(s) to be tested.
▸ Do you want to know what your partner has been up to since their last test?
▸ Do you want to know about your partners' partners?
▸ What kind of barrier use do you want for yourself?
▸ What kind of barrier policies do you want your partners to have with other people?

THE SAFER-SEX TALK

One of the main ways you can mitigate STI risk, along with other sexual-safety risks, is to talk to your partners and potential partners about risk and safety. I'd go so far as to say I think having these talks is essential to a healthy sex life. But I also understand that having these conversations can feel scary. It can help if you have a solid idea of what you want to talk about before you launch into the conversation.

Having a script in mind will help you know what you want to say, what questions you want to ask, and what answers to those questions are acceptable.

You need to decide when and how you feel best having the discussion. "Don't negotiate naked" is a good rule to live by. When sex is imminent, there's too much incentive to hurry through the talk or skip it altogether. So whenever possible, start this conversation in advance. That can mean via text or email before a date, or while you're out in public together. For some, that just means on the couch before you get to the bedroom, or before clothes come off.

Make it clear early on that sexual safety is important to you so that the conversation doesn't feel like it's coming out of the blue. From there, you just need to decide on your own style or what you're comfortable with.

Here are some things you might like to know about potential partners:

- ▸ When were they last tested for STIs?
- ▸ What were they tested for? Saying "everything" doesn't count. Different doctors and clinics have different standard panels, so it's important to ask for details.
- ▸ What were their results?
- ▸ How many partners have they had since their last test?
- ▸ What are their barrier-use practices?

▸ Do they have these talks with all of their partners?
▸ If applicable, what birth control method are they using?

It can be helpful to share this information about yourself first and then ask your partner to reciprocate. That way you've opened the door to being vulnerable, and you've also modeled what you'd like to hear. It tends to work like magic. Although you might need to prompt if something you care about wasn't covered, most people will mirror what you've said and share the same information.

When I'm initiating the talk, I tend to keep it fairly simple so that having the safety talk seems casual and natural, rather than a point of stress. I've often opened the topic via text already, but if I've gotten as far as making out with someone and things seem to be progressing, I'll simply pause and say, "Can we have a chat?" For people who are used to safer-sex talks, they'll usually know what comes next. Generally I'll just launch into my own information: "I was last tested X months ago. I was tested for . . . and the results were . . . I've had X partners since my last test and we've used barriers for penetration, but not always for oral sex." Whenever I'm done sharing my information, I end by saying, "What about you?" This indicates I'd like the same information from them.

Reid Mihalko, who coined the Safer Sex Elevator Speech, also suggests adding one thing you do like and one thing you don't like sexually to the end of the chat, to help facilitate a transition into the rest of your negotiations.

Keep in mind that not everyone is used to having these talks. Some people may never have had them at all. So you might need to do some teaching or offer some guidance to get them used to the process.

A note on language—you may be used to hearing, or even saying, "clean" to mean negative test results. Although that might be a reflexive comment, think about what that's saying. The opposite of clean is dirty, which suggests people with an STI are dirty. There are some STIs people live with their whole lives that can be well managed, and others people may have had and been treated for. Suggesting that someone is dirty for having an STI contributes to stigma and makes it less likely people will be willing to have these conversations, making everyone less safe.

When it comes to barriers, most people are used to condoms for penetrative sex. But what about dental dams? Or gloves? This is another area where you'll need to educate yourself around safety, so you can decide what practices you're most comfortable with for your own sex life and what you want your partners to be doing, or to have done, with their previous partners.

Just as important as the answers to these questions is *how* someone has this conversation. It's true that some people may be taken off guard because they've never been asked about sexual safety before. But if someone seems angry, defensive, or evasive, that's a red flag. I've heard people say, "Don't you trust me?" And the answer is no, not if you can't have this conversation.

When someone is clearly comfortable having the conversation, that's a clue that they've done it before, and it's even more likely that they're talking to other partners about sexual-safety issues. These cues shouldn't replace an explicit conversation, but they can be important hints as to how someone views safety issues.

If you've already set the precedent that you talk about things to do with sex and relationships, it shouldn't come out of the blue when you want to talk about safety, too. And having this conversation before sex also makes it easier to transition into conversations about what kind of sex you'd like to have. After all, once you've done the stuff that feels scary, the rest is a piece of cake.

FLUID BONDING

Fluid bonding, generally, refers to people who have unprotected sex, and therefore share fluids. You'll most often hear this term thrown around in open relationship communities, but it may come up with anyone who is sexually active. The term itself can be complicated, because people use it in different ways. Some people only mean penis-in-vagina sex; others are including oral sex. Yet other people take issue with the concept because they feel fluid bonding is used to designate priority, or that people use the added risk they're taking on to control a partner's other behaviors or choices. Politics aside, you should know that choosing to forgo barriers for oral or penetrative sex does expose you to more risk, and if you're going to go there with someone, it should be someone you trust.

If you want to have a conversation about fluid bonding with a partner, you should give yourself plenty of time. Don't expect to come to any decisions in just one chat. Give yourself time to think about it, and process your feelings on the subject, and to come back and ask questions.

If you and/or your partner have other partners, you should discuss this topic with them as well, as it could expose them to additional risk. And if there's someone you have sex with, without the use of barriers, this should also be something you disclose to new potential partners.

If you want to dig into the relationship politics piece, check out some of the books on open relationships from the resources section.

9   Difficult Conversations

HOW TO GIVE AND ACCEPT AN APOLOGY

Everyone makes mistakes at some point. How you handle it and if—and how—you apologize can make a big difference. We've all experienced it—the apology that makes us even angrier rather than making the situation better. A personal pet peeve is when an apology comes in the form of, "Well, I'm sorry you feel that way." Phrasing it in those terms doesn't take any responsibility for what's happened.

So how do you apologize well?

First, we need to get over the guilt or embarrassment that makes us want to ignore the situation and move on. And while the urge to hide your head in the sand is totally understandable, ultimately it'll make things worse and potentially even destroy the relationship.

It's important to have an understanding of what happened. Perhaps you've heard the saying that the best apology is changed behavior? Well, you can't make changes if you don't know what went wrong. So the first step has to be a conversation with the other person so you can both come to an understanding of what happened and why.

Another saying is that apologies don't come with buts. The idea is that if you're making an excuse (even if you think it's an explanation) in the same breath as the apology, then the apology probably won't mean much. This doesn't mean you don't want to figure out what factors led to the situation, but that conversation needs to be separate from the apology.

An effective apology needs to acknowledge the hurt that was caused. People want to know that their partner sees the harm that was done. Without this piece, it will seem like the person apologizing doesn't think it's a big deal, and it's harder to believe the apology is sincere and that the incident won't happen again.

Even when there's been a sincere apology, hurt feelings can linger. It's important to give someone a chance to process and heal. The time it takes could be anywhere from minutes to days, maybe even weeks or more, depending on the amount of hurt that was caused.

However, once an apology has been given and accepted, try to let go as much as possible, and don't bring up the incident every time there's a fight. While it's important to see patterns of behavior because sometimes they indicate a relationship isn't healthy, it also creates a bigger divide to recite a litany of grievances whenever there's an upset.

The most effective apologies involve taking responsibility for your actions, or for whatever hurtful thing happened. None of us ever wants to be the bad guy, so you might need to take a minute with this one and admit to yourself that you screwed up, so you can admit it to your partner.

You also want to apologize as soon as possible. The longer it takes to acknowledge what happened, the harder it will be to make amends. You leave your partner wondering if you understand that something hurtful happened and give them more time to stew in their feelings.

Next up, how will you make it right? Sometimes it's just the apology that's needed, and sometimes there are tangible steps that can be taken. The person apologizing can make an offer, or they can simply ask the other party what they need.

When you're apologizing, make sure to keep the focus on the person who was harmed. Sometimes we feel so bad about what happened, it's easy to tip over into saying things like, "I'm the worst partner." Even if you're feeling that way in the moment, keep in mind that expressing that shifts the focus to you and puts your partner in a position of having to comfort you rather than feeling comforted themselves.

One of the reasons that apologies are so important is that they help restore trust. Without an apology, it can seem like both parties don't agree on whether something went wrong. And the person who feels hurt has no assurances that the same thing won't happen again. This feeling is always a problem that can eat at a relationship, but it can be especially damaging in sex and kink, where a lack of trust or sense of safety can completely derail the activities you'd like to engage in.

For this reason, it's helpful if an apology can include a promise that the same thing won't happen again. Be careful with this one—don't make this promise if it's not something you believe you can follow through on. Having the same thing happen again, especially after a promise, can irreparably harm a relationship.

THE EX TALK

When I'm getting to know someone new, one of the first things I look out for is how they talk about their exes. Are they still friends or do they have a lot of complaints about people they used to date? Even worse, do they tell you about how "crazy" an ex was?

Sure, most of us have had one or two relationships that weren't so great, with people we don't care to stay friends with. But if someone has a long string of disaster stories, you've got to notice that it's the person talking who is the common thread.

Not just that, but look at the language someone uses when talking about other people. Are they dismissive or sex negative in some way? Do they use terms like *slut* when describing people? (Assuming they're not using it in an empowered, reclaimed way.) Some people have a pattern of going through partners and convincing themselves that their partners were the problem. You'll save yourself some time and heartache if you avoid those folks.

Beyond how they talk about partners, how do they talk about their friends? Or even celebrities? Do they use body-shaming or judgmental language? All of these things are clues to how this person will ultimately treat you.

Assuming there are no glaring red flags, talking about past relationships can be a great way to get to know someone.

We can learn a lot about someone by hearing about the relationships they've been in.

Like we talked about in the section on sharing secrets in chapter 6, it's important to set parameters for these conversations. How much information do you really want? Sometimes it's best to get a general overview, rather than a play-by-play. How people met, how long they were together, and maybe why they broke up can be good starting points.

When it's done well, having this conversation can be a good way to not only share personal information but share being vulnerable, and that can help build trust and bring you closer together. Also, sometimes talking about your past relationships can help you see some of the reasons they didn't work, and help you avoid those pitfalls in the future.

ATTRACTION TO OTHER PEOPLE

Even if we've committed to a monogamous relationship, we still find other people attractive. Monogamy is an agreement about actions, not thoughts. But all too often we put our partners in a position of having to lie to us by acting like attraction is a thought crime.

In some relationships, everything from porn to looking at someone walking down the street gets policed. In fact, when I'm teaching in colleges, I'm often asked if watching porn or masturbating is considered cheating.

When I was in a monogamous marriage, my partner and I talked about our attractions. From movie stars to people we worked with, we openly acknowledged when we thought someone was hot. It became almost a game. And it also brought us closer because we were learning things about each other during these conversations, and also proving that it was safe to be vulnerable in that way.

Like we talked about in the section on game playing, it's not healthy to try to "test" your partner. This comes up in the attraction arena with some frequency, with asking their partner if they find someone attractive, only to pounce on them if the answer is yes.

Don't ask a question you don't want an answer to, and don't put your partner in a situation where they have to lie to you. If you make it unsafe to be attracted to other people, you're creating secrets in your relationship.

If you're going to have an open conversation about attraction to other people, remember it doesn't need to be an explicit rundown. You don't need to detail someone's every amazing quality, and you most certainly don't want to compare them to your partner.

Instead, keep it academic and simple, just stating a fact. If you're able to have these conversations in a neutral way, you may be able to get to know your partner better and learn new things about their interests.

MISMATCHED DESIRE

Perhaps few things are as confusing as our culture's idea of how much sex you're supposed to want to have. Too much and you're a slut. Too little and you're frigid. Where are the lines? No one knows. And these biases are highly gendered as well. Basically no one comes out a winner. Instead, we're all left worrying if there's something wrong with us, or if we'll be judged by our peers.

No wonder then that asking for sex can be a touchy

subject. If we feel bad for not wanting sex when our partner does, it can be a knee-jerk reaction to judge them for being insatiable, rather than to calmly recognize that there's a simple mismatch in interest or desire. Likewise, if we ask for sex and are denied, it can be easy to think of our partner as lacking passion or feeling for us.

Not only do different people have different levels of interest in sex, but these levels can change many times over the course of our lives. And many of us are unprepared for those changes. Whether due to lifestyle changes, parenthood, work stress, or simply change over time, we often expect our bodies to be fixed in their prime, and the reality just isn't so.

Some people are in relationships where there has always been a mismatch in desired frequency. For others, one person's interest changes over time. Either can be frustrating—especially if there isn't clear communication around the subject.

Sometimes a partner's actions make us less interested in having sex with them. Whether it's something in the relationship that makes us less happy or less comfortable, or something about the sexual encounters we have, it needs to be addressed.

Even if the actual problems aren't fun to talk about, our minds tend to concoct worst-case scenarios that are even worse than the truth. And thinking our partners no longer desire us can eat away at all aspects of a relationship.

However, with touchy subjects, talking isn't always easy. When we're embarrassed, or when we feel judged, our reactions can be less than levelheaded. And so much ego is tied up in our perceived desirability. But left unaddressed, a mismatch in sexual desire is an issue that will fester.

First, it's worth determining if there are factors contributing to lower desire that can be addressed. If you're cranky that your partner isn't helping with the housework, say so. It might still be an uncomfortable conversation, but it's one you can get through. If your reluctance is about how the sex itself is going, that's important to share, too. If you're not getting pleasure from sex, address that issue head-on rather than avoiding sex. As hard as the conversations may be to have, they're better than a relationship that slowly drifts apart.

When you have a conversation about the mismatch, it's important to frame it with the understanding that there's nothing wrong with either one of you. "Normal" really isn't a helpful concept when it comes to sexuality, and there's a wide range of natural and healthy ways to be.

Further complicating the issue, many people feel validated by being desired sexually, so when their partners don't want sex, their confidence can really take a hit. That's part of why it's so important to handle the situation with empathy and delicacy. If the lack of desire is simply that, a lack of desire, and not indicative of household, relationship, or sexual problems, it's important to say so.

While less sex is happening, it's important to make sure you still have other forms of intimacy. Find ways to spend quality time together, have deep conversations, and have nonsexual touch like snuggling. This often stops happening, along with sex, because the partner who is less interested in sex gets worried about leading the other person on and then saying no. And they end up turning down other basic forms of connection like cuddling or massage. It can be extremely valuable to have an open conversation about this to make sure all your chances for intimacy and connection don't evaporate while you're juggling varying levels of interest in sex.

Like so many things, this conversation is best had as simply and directly as possible. You could say, "Hey, I don't feel like having sex tonight, but I'd really love to snuggle for a while." Just substitute whatever activity you'd like to engage in—maybe playing a game, or showering together, or whatever else makes you feel close.

It's also helpful to have an explicit understanding that it's okay to ask for sex without shame, and equally okay to turn it down without shame. This might not be as easy as it sounds if sex has already become a loaded subject, but getting back to a place where you can discuss it matter-of-factly can be a huge help.

When you're looking for ways to get everyone's needs met, see if there are ways to reach a win-win agreement. Perhaps the partner who wants sex can masturbate while the other partner snuggles or touches them—that can be a great way to compromise.

Sex is important to many people's well-being, and if a mismatch in desire remains long term, it could be time to look at other options. Sometimes an open relationship is a good way to let someone get their needs met elsewhere. You can also seek guidance from a couples' counselor or sex coach. (See the resources section for tips on how to find help—and check out Emily Nagoski's book *Come as You Are*.)

HOW TO FIGHT FAIR

Every relationship will have a conflict at some point. What matters is how you handle it. Conflicts can be a great test of a relationship because being able to treat each other with kindness and empathy even when tempers flare is essential to long-term harmony.

Especially when a fight comes up in the sexual realm, we can feel sensitive and defensive. The more vulnerable we feel when something goes wrong, the trickier it might be. So in order to try more intensely intimate sex acts, or riskier kink activities, we've got to have strong conflict-resolution skills.

First up is owning your own feelings and not assigning blame. When possible, talk about the problem, not the person. It's not "you're a terrible partner," it's "when this thing happens, I feel hurt." (For more on using "I" statements, reread that section of chapter 6.)

Where possible, assume innocence or good intentions unless proven otherwise. In a healthy relationship, it's more likely something was an accident, or a miscommunication, than something done to intentionally hurt you. Let the other person speak their piece, and together you can figure out what went wrong and how to keep it from happening again.

Fights get dirty when we lay blame, call names, bring up past conflicts, raise our voices, or speak in mocking or aggressive tones. Using these tactics will only make things worse rather than working toward resolution.

As much as possible, stay in touch with your feelings and know when you need to pause or take a break. There comes a point when emotions are running so high that productive conversation is no longer likely to take place.

Avoid making generalizations like "you always . . ." or "you never . . ." It can be frustrating when we sense a pattern, but making accusations, especially sweeping ones, will likely put the other person on the defensive. And that's not a great position for either of you to be in if you want to resolve the issue at hand.

When we're upset and having a difficult conversation, sometimes we start listing all the things that upset us. This kind of piling on tends to derail a conversation. I'm not saying that each thing that upsets you isn't valid, but they'll each need to have their own conversation. When you're trying to resolve a conflict, pick just one issue or topic at a time, and then take a good break before the next difficult conversation. Make sure to focus on positive time together, and intimacy building, so you're back to a solid base from which to have the next difficult conversation.

ADMITTING YOU'VE LIED

Most of the tools in this book will help you have a better, more pleasurable sex life. And while talking about sex with your partner might feel tricky at first if you haven't been in that habit, most couples can accept that there's always some room for improvement.

But what if you've been lying? What if you've been saying that you love the sex you're having, or you've been faking orgasms? Or what if you haven't said anything, and you've just let your partner think you enjoy everything that's happening, but really you're considering the shopping list, or counting down time until you're done? In these cases, you're going to need to come clean, and you're going to have to be gentle doing it.

Having this conversation means the double whammy of making it clear you haven't been honest while also explaining you're not enjoying sex. The person hearing these things will likely feel hurt. You don't want to compound the issue with more lies, but you can be gentle and thoughtful about how you have the conversation.

If you've been faking orgasms, the good news—or bad news, depending on how you look at it—is that you're not alone. Although the numbers vary, studies show that a significant percentage of people are faking orgasms (or not correcting partners who think they've had an orgasm) or are lying about sexual pleasure in general.

Because this is such a touchy subject, it's best to employ all the techniques we've discussed for how to have tricky or vulnerable conversations. For one, you don't want to do this during sex, or while one or both of you is naked. This is a conversation best had with clothes on, in a space where everyone feels secure, either at home or in a public place with plenty of privacy. Maybe even on a walk. Sometimes movement, like walking, can help facilitate conversations.

You also don't want to surprise your partner with this conversation. Let them know you want to talk about something sensitive, and let them opt in to the conversation. You want to make sure to pick a time that they're ready for it. Just like scheduling any other important talk, you want to make sure everyone is well rested, well fed, and in a good mood.

When it's time for the talk, you want to focus on "I" statements. You're making this about you, not accusations that your partner is lousy in bed. In fact, that's exactly the assumption you're trying to avoid. As much as possible, explain why you haven't been honest. Have you felt frustrated or self-conscious about your body, or how your body performs sexually? Were you afraid your partner would be less into you if it was more difficult for you to orgasm?

Not only that, but tell your partner how you feel about having this conversation. Are you nervous? Scared? Tell them that. And tell them what you need in order to get through the conversation. Maybe ask them to just listen and not ask questions until you're done. Whatever it takes for you to say what you need to say.

Many of us have been socialized to think it's not okay to be too much work. We want to be easy. Easy to love, easy to live with, and easy to pleasure. When these messages are internalized, faking orgasms is one of the ways that pressure can manifest.

You'll have to do some thinking on your own to come up with all the reasons you haven't been honest, but if you can share those reasons in a genuine and vulnerable way, hopefully your partner can empathize with your situation rather than focusing on their own bruised ego.

Another technique we've talked about before that you'll want to employ here is focusing on the positive. Before you drop the bomb (and even during and after), make sure you're also saying what you do enjoy about your sex and intimacy. Maybe you really enjoy how your partner touches you. Maybe you enjoy how safe you feel. Maybe the way they kiss is incredible. You can also tell them nonsexual things you enjoy about the relationship. I'm not suggesting disingenuous ego stroking, but find things you really do enjoy that you can talk about.

When you start exploring ways to have orgasms together, be ready to make suggestions. Don't just say that what's been happening isn't working and then leave your partner to figure out another plan. Instead, be ready to show them exactly what works. Ideally you've figured out how to have orgasms on your own, so you can show your partner what you like. If you're also not having orgasms by yourself, that's something worth sharing with your partner and probably the first thing to work on.

As for suggestions, if you usually masturbate with a sex toy, try bringing that sex toy into your partnered play. Do what you know works while your partner is there to participate. Also be ready to make other concrete suggestions, like changing the way someone holds their hand, how many fingers they use to touch you, at what pace they're moving . . . anything you can do that will give them guidance about what you like.

If coming right out and saying you've lied or faked feels impossible, all is not lost. While I think honesty is the best policy, I understand why in this case people might be unwilling to go there. If you're not having orgasms, or simply not having much sexual pleasure, you can still adjust your sex life without saying you're not enjoying yourself now.

Focus on trying new things, experiencing new sensations, or talking about more intense pleasure. If you've been primarily focusing on external pleasure (penis, clitoris) try exploring internal stimulation (prostate, G-spot). This way you can start finding new ways to enjoy yourself before you start modifying the existing ways you're playing. And once you've had some fun exploring new things, it might be easier to say, "If there's so much pleasure here we didn't know about, I wonder what else we can discover!"

Exploring things like slow sex, orgasmic meditation, and tantra are all ways you can introduce things that are new enough it can feel like starting from scratch, without making it clear that what you were doing before was a bust.

Finally, it's important to remember that your sexual pleasure matters! Life is too short to not explore all the pleasure that's available to you. Sometimes it'll feel hard, but I promise that it's worth pushing through the difficult moments to see what experiences are possible.

HOW TO BREAK UP WITH SOMEONE

Breakups. Most people have had at least one. Some of us have had several. In one of the most regrettable moments of my life, I once broke up with someone by sliding a note into their locker. (I was thirteen.) To this day I feel awful about that. Even though we'd only been on one real date, he deserved to hear it from me face-to-face. But I was young, inexperienced (he was my first kiss), and terrified of having to face his reaction. Hence, the note. These days perhaps that doesn't sound so shocking. In the age of ghosting, maybe getting a note sounds pretty good.

Although I'm not one to bemoan the ways technology is breaking down human interaction (you'll never catch me shaming someone for looking at their phone), I do think dating apps are making it a bit too easy to treat people as disposable.

Some articles have come out in favor of ghosting, arguing that just disappearing is preferable to a direct rejection, but I couldn't disagree more. I don't want those open questions left in my mind. If something is over, even if it's a conversation that never led to a meeting, I want to know it.

Of course, there are some good reasons people don't give direct rejections. Online, people sometimes become hostile when faced with rejection. In person, it can be even scarier. So if you need to be vague or say "maybe" for your safety, do so. But when possible, direct communication is best.

So how do you break up with someone? This is a situation where "do unto others" comes into play. How would you want someone to break up with you? For me, I think being kind is paramount. And rely on the things we've talked about already. Let someone know you need to talk, and choose a neutral, maybe public, location. It can help to have an outline of what you want to say. You can have actual notes if you think you'll need them, but at a minimum have an idea of the points you need to cover.

When you're breaking up with someone, it's not a negotiation. You're always allowed to leave a relationship for any reason. So don't feel pressured to try again or make compromises. This is also your chance to set boundaries about what you need moving forward. If you need a break before you start talking to this person again or start trying to be friends, it's okay to say so. Sometimes taking a break is the best way to take time to heal so that you can salvage a friendship a few weeks or months down the line.

I don't consider breakups failures. Sometimes people simply aren't right for each other anymore, and it doesn't have to be anyone's fault, or because anything terrible happened. It's okay, and often valuable, to acknowledge the good things from the relationship—what you learned, what you experienced, fond memories you have. Sometimes you still love the person you're breaking up with. Keeping it positive, when appropriate, can also set the tone for a future friendship.

Breakups come in many forms. I'm using the term loosely here. It can certainly mean ending a relationship. But it could also mean other kinds of endings. Maybe you've realized that someone you've been doing kink play with for a while isn't a good fit anymore. Or you need to end things with someone who has been a casual sex friend. The less involved a connection was, the more tempting it can be to just disappear on someone, but I don't think that models the direct and honest communication we're striving for here.

Perhaps this is overly optimistic of me, but I think good communication isn't just about our lives and our relationships, but also about modeling best practices so that people will go out in the world and do better. I think we can actually create a culture shift with good communication. That's how I sometimes encourage myself to have hard conversations I'm tempted to avoid. I ask myself what kind of world I want to live in—a world where people talk about the hard stuff openly and with compassion? Or a world where we take the easy road for ourselves at the cost of other people's feelings? When I put it that way, it's an easy choice.

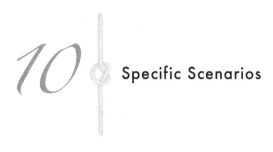

10 Specific Scenarios

GETTING INVITED
WHETHER IT'S FROM FRIENDS, CLIENTS, OR students, one of the most common questions I'm asked is how to make threesomes happen and/or how to get invited to sex parties. Sometimes it's as easy as creating a profile on an app that puts like-minded people together for such things, but more often it's mingling with the right people and showing your ability to handle these situations.

I was recently on a date with a couple I'd met online. This is something I rarely do, not because I'm opposed to being a unicorn, but because these meetings with strangers rarely go well. An online date with a stranger is already a crapshoot, but with a couple you need to like both of them, and like their dynamic with each other.

So while I have lots of threesomes and group sex, it's generally with people who are already my friends and lovers. People I've already cultivated trust with. People I know are on the same page as me with safety and who can communicate about their needs and limits.

As I talked with this couple over a drink, the thing that impressed me the most was the way they behaved with each other. Not only were they stopping to check in with each other on a regular basis, but the stories they told me about their play with other couples demonstrated the ways they were looking out for each other and themselves.

I ended up going home with them. Yes, they were both attractive. But what really sold me was that I knew I could trust them to communicate clearly with me. I felt confident that I wouldn't end up in the middle of a fight between them because someone crossed a boundary or got their feelings hurt. Not only that, but when I made it clear I was only comfortable with hand sex, they didn't complain for an instant but fully embraced the play I was willing to do.

This whole experience hinged on open, honest, and clear communication. And as you've likely gathered by now, I think that's what all good sex comes from.

So one of the best things you can do to get yourself in these situations is to start meeting people who already engage in the activities you're interested in, and then show that you're trustworthy and a good communicator. If you're interested in meeting kinky folks, look for your local munches. A munch is a gathering of kinky people in a vanilla environment, like a bar or restaurant. They get the name *munch* because they're usually held somewhere food is served. You can also find mixers and meet-ups for other specific communities, like swingers or polyamorous folks. Whatever group you go to, make sure you get to know people as people. Show that you're interested in them, and in the community, and that you're not simply on the hunt for someone to fulfill a fantasy.

Those of us who are veterans of these communities can tell in an instant who is treating people as disposable and who is genuinely interested in not just the experience, but the people having it.

THREESOMES

Like so many things to do with sex, people want three-somes to just happen organically or spontaneously. But even when that's what seems to be happening, there's more going on under the surface. Threesomes take planning and negotiation, especially when it's the first time for this combination of people—even if all the people have slept together separately before. Each person involved needs to be clear about what they want from the experience, and what boundaries they have.

I always advocate having your negotiations well in advance of the proposed play, and I think that's especially important for threesomes or group play. When there's an audience, or people you're less familiar with, it can be harder to speak up in the moment. So do as much talking in advance as you can, but still check in when you all get together.

Here are some specific considerations.

Safer Sex

▸ Safer sex always needs to be on your negotiation list, but with threesomes it's even more essential to cover in advance, because when there are more bodies, and new experiences, it's easy to get carried away and forget to check in.

▸ In addition to your usual safer-sex conversation, there are some additional considerations for threesomes/group sex. For one, you'll need to mind your fluids even more carefully than usual, especially if you have different limits for different people.

▸ Gloves can be a great way to keep fluids contained. Even if you wouldn't usually use them for one-on-one sex, in threesomes they can be a huge help. With gloves, you can color code whom you're touching with what hand, and you can change out gloves as needed for a clean slate.

▸ You also need to pay attention to where your mouth goes. Going directly from one person's genitals to another's can transmit anything hands or direct contact can, so if everyone doesn't want to share fluids or skin contact, sometimes it's easier to simply skip oral.

▸ Another option if you can be disciplined about it is to wash up between partners. Don't brush your teeth, because that will cause microtears in your gums (and maybe even draw blood), but you can wash your face off with soap and water and rinse your mouth with mouthwash. Unfortunately the studies are limited, but there is some evidence that mouthwash can provide limited protection against certain infections.[7]

---

7   Eric P. F. Chow, et al., "Antiseptic Mouthwash Against Pharyngeal *Neisseria gonorrhoeae*: A Randomised Controlled Trial and an In Vitro Study," *Sexually Transmitted Infections* 93, no. 2 (17 February 2017): 88–93. http://sti.bmj.com/lookup/doi/10.1136/sextrans-2016-052753.

An established couple adding a third

▸ When there's an established couple, they need to have their own negotiation in addition to negotiating with the new person. Do your relationship boundaries include any acts that are only for the two of you? Are there limits to what you want to do with a new person?

▸ Threesomes are a common fantasy, but not everyone thinks through the possible consequences. How do you think you'll really feel watching your partner kiss, or have sex with, another person? Will you think it's hot, or will it make you sad or jealous?

▸ Sometimes finding baby steps toward a threesome is the best way to start—maybe going to a strip club together, so you can watch your partner flirt, or be flirted with. Maybe watch them get a private dance. How does it feel for them to look at, and be aroused by, another person? This can give you clues about how you'll feel in a threesome, and if it's something you're ready for.

▸ Make sure you're treating your third like a person, not a sex toy. (Unless that's their kink!) This means that you acknowledge they have their own reasons for joining you, and their own wants and desires for the encounter. Make sure you ask what they're hoping to get out of the experience, and what kind of aftercare they're looking for. Is this a onetime thing? Is it the beginning of an occasional, casual relationship? Something more? Make sure everyone has the same expectations, to avoid hurt feelings.

▸ What about spending the night? Some couples expect to spend the night just the two of them, as a chance to reconnect after the threesome. If that's your plan, make sure you talk to your third about it in advance, so you're not kicking them out after sex, when they're grabbing their toothbrush and jammies.

For everyone

▸ Think about what you're hoping to get from this experience, and especially if it's your first threesome, be realistic. For first-time play, it can be great to start with snuggles, make outs, or massages. There's no reason you need to have nudity or sex to get a thrill out of adding a person to your play. And starting with these other activities can be a great way to get used to negotiating with a new person, before the stakes are too high.

▸ What happens if someone needs to step out of the room? Does all play stop until they get back, or do you continue and let them join back in when they return?

▸ Think about how everyone's sexuality and attraction align. The most common threesome fantasy you see in media involves a unicorn—a bisexual woman who's equally attracted to both people in the typically cis hetero/flexible couple. But that's not how it has to look.

▸ Decide on what threesome configuration you're aiming for. Sometimes one person is the center of attention, and sometimes all the people are equally involved. Any configuration you can imagine is fine, as long as that's what everyone is signing up for. Be sure to talk about this in advance, so there aren't hurt feelings in the middle of play.

Performance issues

▸ Bodies are unpredictable and don't always perform exactly how you'd like them to—especially under pressure. Be prepared to be flexible about what activities you're going to do, and be ready to improvise with sex toys. If, for example, your fantasy is double penetration with two bio cocks, remember that coordinating erections isn't as easy as it looks in porn. Toys can be a blessing in these circumstances, because they're always ready to go.

▸ If someone finds they can't do the things they'd planned on, be gentle with them. This is a vulnerable position to be in, so it's important to be mindful of everyone's feelings. How you deal with these kinds of issues will be a consideration for whether the same people will want to play with you again.

▸ As with all things sex related, having an open mind, and not being goal oriented, will serve you well in threesomes. While it's great to talk about your fantasies and ideas you'd like to try, make sure you also have several backup plans—including just snuggling.

Aftercare

▸ Aftercare is most commonly talked about in kink, but it's vital for a variety of situations. The idea of aftercare is simply taking extra good care of yourself and/or your partner after you've engaged in something intense. Whenever you try something new, or something that's emotionally vulnerable, make sure to go easy on yourself afterward, as well as check in with your partner(s) about their needs. (Learn more about aftercare in chapter 11.)

▸ If there's an existing couple as part of the three-some, have a check-in with all three participants, as well as planned time to reconnect one on one.

▸ Be sure to check in with your third and see how they're feeling the next day, or a few days later. Sometimes getting together for coffee to check in face-to-face can be really helpful.

▸ If you'd like to get together with the same people again (or just want to learn from this experience), have a conversation about what went well about this threesome and what you might like to improve on for next time.

Follow-ups and check-ins

▸ After any kind of vulnerable or intense play, a follow-up is a great idea. And threesomes can qualify as both vulnerable and intense! Depending on the relationships between the people involved, a simple text the next day might do the trick. Ask how the other person is feeling, see if they need anything, and be sure to thank them for sharing themselves with you!

▸ If things were especially intense, or anything happened that not everyone is feeling good about, getting together in person might be ideal.

▸ Postplay follow-ups are also a great time to discuss what went well, or to express interest in meeting up again sometime.

Don't forget that anyone can tap out at any time! Three-somes can bring up feelings you weren't expecting, even if you've done this before, and it's important that everyone feels comfortable stopping at any time. If this happens, it might be best if all the play stops for the night. Have a contingency plan in advance, like snuggling and watching a movie, so that there's still a way to have connection even if you're not having sex.

Lastly, have fun! A willingness to be silly is key for most sex, and this is doubly (triply?) true when there are more people involved.

I had a personal experience that helped prove three-way play can be hot and exciting without nudity or overt sex acts. A friend of mine who's known for their sex parties invited me to an event, and I made the sponta-neous decision to hop on a plane and attend. I was just visiting for twenty-four hours, and I was excited to see some old friends and to meet a lot of new faces.

These parties always start with an opening circle that goes over the culture of the event and expectations around consent and safety. It also allows people to say a little about what kinds of things they like and what they're hoping to experience for the evening.

After the opening circle, a woman came up to me and asked if we could kiss. I said yes, and after kissing she told me she'd never kissed another woman before. It would have been nice to know that in advance, but I still felt flattered that I seemed like a safe person to her. I asked her why she chose me, and she said I seemed like someone who would take rejection well if she wasn't into it after one kiss. That may seem like a strange thing to say, but I actually thought that was a very good compliment. And I think that's something you should be screening partners for, especially when you're trying something new.

Before long, it came up that she'd never done three-way play, either, and I entered into negotiations with her partner, too. After coming to some basic agreements, we started taking turns making out and touching each other, and then I'd check in with her about how she was doing. Sometimes she was doing great and wanted to keep going, and sometimes she wanted to take a little break. Those breaks sometimes involved us all sitting and chatting, and sometimes she'd go for a little walk or get a snack and then come back.

After maybe forty minutes of this, she said she thought she was done for the night. Her partner didn't hear this, or wasn't listening, because he continued touching me and was trying to negotiate more sexual activity. I had to reiterate what she'd said, that we were done for the night.

This ended up being a good experience for everyone involved, and it was a good example of first time three-way play just involving kissing and touching over clothes. For someone's first time (not to mention their first sex party), that's still a really big step. And it was a much better idea to stop there than to feel like more had to happen, only to risk regretting it later.

It's also an example of how important communication is during a threesome—including communication between partners. It's easy for someone to get carried away, or to have a particular goal in mind that they're pushing for. But being goal oriented in that way makes it easy for disappointment or hurt feelings to happen.

Like with all things to do with sex, approaching

threesomes with an open mind is the best way to have a good experience.

GROUP SEX/PARTIES

From events at public venues to private house parties, there are lots of opportunities to get your sex or kink on in a public or semipublic space. Some people enjoy the voyeurism or exhibitionism aspect; others enjoy the safety of having bystanders and party hosts on hand to help if things go sideways. Parties can also offer access to specific equipment, from dungeon furniture to sex swings, so you can play in ways that might not be feasible at home. Parties can also be good places to meet playmates, either for one-on-one play or for threesomes and group play.

When you're planning to check out a new party or venue, it's important to find out both the culture and the rules of the space. Being on top of your communication skills is always a great idea, and it's essential in these scenarios. From how to negotiate play with new people, to negotiating boundaries with existing partners, there's more to think about at parties than on a one-on-one date.

Going to a kink or sex party is such a unique experience that things are bound to come up that you haven't thought of in your usual relationship negotiations, even if you've had threesomes before.

First of all, if you're going to the party with a partner, you'll want to look over all of the details of the event together. Read the venue and event rules, everything from dress code to substance use. Try to anticipate what the night will include so that you can have discussions and negotiations in advance. And also plan for how to check in on the fly.

Remember, just because you're at a party doesn't mean you have to play. Whether solo or with a partner, just going to watch is totally okay! After all, the exhibitionists need an audience, and voyeurism is participation.

Here are some specific things to consider.

Substance use
If it's at a public club, there might be a bar. At a private home, sometimes drinks are served. Will you or your partner drink? If so, how much? Are you willing to play with people who have been drinking? It's common to see people using alcohol to relax and get comfortable, but that's got a big downside. Substance use means impaired judgment—it's just a matter of degree. So make sure you know yourself and your limits, and make a plan in advance about if, and how much, you're going to drink.

Outfits and packing
Talk about what you're going to wear and what you're going to bring. Are you bringing toys? If so, are they only for use by you or your partner, or will they be shared with others?

Safer sex
Some events provide their own safer-sex supplies, but it's always a good idea to have your own favorites with you. Some spaces will provide condoms but not gloves or dental dams. So again, it's helpful to have whatever you'd normally use on hand.

Are you going as a date?
If so, what does that mean to you? Are you staying by each

other's sides once you're there, or are you going your own way as free agents, just meeting back up to leave together? Are you playing together or separately? Either way, what kind of check-ins do you want?

If you're planning to play with other people together, it's best to have a check-in with your partner when the other person or people aren't around, to make sure you can speak freely. A common trap is to agree to something because you think it's what your partner wants, only to find out later that you were both doing it for the other person. Don't let that happen to you.

This is important and bears repeating: *Don't do something just because you think the other person or people want it!*

When going to a party with a partner

Try to have two layers of negotiation. One before you leave for the event, where you can talk about what kinds of things you're interested in and what's definitely off the table. And make sure those hard limits are respected in the moment. If you decided that this time you're only going to watch, but then an individual or couple approaches you, stick to your original plan. You can always get their information and hook up another time when you've been able to think and talk about it. But pushing past stated boundaries in the moment, even if it seems like a good idea at the time, is risky.

Then, when you're at the event, make sure you have a protocol for how you'll negotiate in the moment. If someone approaches you and offers something that's within your negotiation, still take a step back to talk about it. Just because you said playing with another couple (for example) was on the table, you still need to make sure both of you are comfortable with *this* couple.

Changing your mind is always an option

If you stop feeling one hundred percent comfortable at any time, you can always stop or change activities. Anyone who gives you a hard time about that isn't someone you should be playing with. If you need to leave early, that's okay. Better to have a short experience and go back another time if you're feeling it than to push past your comfort zone on the first try.

If you're partnered, but going to a party alone

Just because your partner won't be with you at the party doesn't mean you don't have to negotiate. In fact, because they won't be there for check-ins, it can be even more important to make sure you're on the same page ahead of time.

What are your boundaries for the night? Will you be engaging with existing friends and play partners? Will you be playing with new people? What levels of nudity or touch will you engage in? What levels of sex play? What safer-sex barriers will you use?

Also think about what happens when you get home. How will you reconnect? What level of detail will you share about what happened? Sometimes people don't know what they'll need in advance, so if this is a first for you, be prepared to feel some of this out as you go, with lots of check-ins along the way.

How might that look?

Jess walks through the door and drops her bag on the floor. She's exhausted and kicks off her high heels before taking another step into the room. Hearing the door close, Marcus pads into the living room, in his pajamas, to greet her.

"Hey, baby, did you have a fun night?" he asks, giving her a quick hug and a kiss on the cheek.

"I did! Chelsea and Bo met me out front and we spent the first hour just dancing. My feet are killing me. I also played a little—do you want to hear about it?" Jess asks as they move to the couch to sit down.

Marcus thinks for a minute before he answers. "How about just the broad strokes first."

Jess thinks about what information to share and tells him, "David was there, the guy I'd been telling you about? And we slept together." She stops at that, saving the details for if Marcus asks questions.

"That's great. I'm so glad you had a good time," Marcus says, giving Jess another squeeze. They stay like that on the couch for a few minutes, just snuggling each other. "I was half-asleep when I heard you come in. How about we get some sleep and you tell me the rest in the morning?"

"Sounds good," Jess answers, giving his leg a squeeze before standing up to get undressed and ready for bed. When she finally slides under the covers, she feels like she might melt into the comfort of her bed and her partner's arms around her.

They both sleep soundly, knowing they can have the rest of their debriefing over their morning coffee.

After a group-sex experience with one of my partners, he was marveling at how amazing it was to have our connection be seen in that way. Having both friends and strangers witness the vulnerability he and I shared. When I wondered out loud how people who didn't engage in public sex got that kind of validation of their connection, he had an immediate (if tongue-in-cheek) answer: weddings. And while I think that's a bit of a stretch, there's also truth to it. Once you work out the logistics, it can be amazing to celebrate your emotional and sexual connection where other people can witness it.

At the same time, parties are a chance to see the ways other people play. Being in a sexually charged environment can be a great way to get your own juices flowing, as well as get ideas for things you might like to try.

Sadly, there aren't opportunities to learn about sex by watching in most areas of our lives. But sometimes watching is the best way to learn everything from new techniques to whole new acts to try. Going to parties can be a great way to open new doors. And with the right negotiations in place, it can be a smooth and fun experience for everyone.

SUBSTANCE USE

Substance use is a tricky topic, and one that you want to make sure you're addressing before any sex or play happens. Many people want all of their play to be sober, and many others like playing while altered. This can be a serious mismatch. And for yet other people, only light intoxication is acceptable. It's important to negotiate substance use in advance, because when people are impaired, they don't always know how severe it is.

It's common for kink parties to be substance-free, while many sex clubs have bars. So you always need to know the culture, rules, and expectations for venues and events you'd like to attend.

One of the reasons it's vital to consider substance use is because substances can impact a person's ability to give consent. It's not uncommon when people are trying something new—like a first date, a first threesome, or a first sex party—to want a little social lubricant. But everyone reacts to substances differently, and while one person might be fine having a glass of wine and then making decisions about risky behavior, other people might do things they'll later regret.

If the risks around consent aren't enough to give you pause, keep in mind that many substances, including alcohol and even pot, can affect both levels of desire and your body's ability to perform. Not only that, but they can affect your relationship with pain, too, and that can make things tricky if you're playing with kink. Using a substance that dulls your pain response might feel great in the moment, but you could wake up with a lot more bruises and soreness than you bargained for.

Although I strongly encourage you to have your new encounters while sober, at a minimum make sure you have your negotiations, and set your boundaries, well before any substance use takes place.

FIRST DATES

First dates—you either love them or hate them. There's a question on OKCupid about whether first dates or job interviews make you more nervous, and I've always thought that's very telling about a person. Personally I'm not a first-date fan. I prefer the juicy stuff after intimacy and connection have been established.

But first dates go a lot more smoothly when you've got communication skills to rely on, and when you're comfortable negotiating. Everything from planning where to go to greetings and good-nights, from deciding who pays to checking in about how things went and whether there will be a second date, comes down to communication and negotiation.

A common question in my Modern Dating class is how to greet people at the beginning of a date and how to say good night at the end. People are expecting me to tell them something like, "All dates start with a hug and end with a kiss." But of course it's not that simple. The only answer is to ask the other person. Are you a person who likes to give hugs? Then at the beginning of the date, when you meet the other person, ask if you can hug them. That's the easiest way to know if someone wants something—ask them.

The same is true for the end of the night—if you want a good-night kiss, say so. Maybe you aren't even waiting until the end of the night—maybe something they said or the way the light hits their face makes you want to kiss them during the date. Say so!

People worry that talking ruins the mood, but that's rarely true if it's done well. You just need to integrate it into your style. So if you're sitting watching the sunset with someone and their face is glowing in the reflection and looks especially beautiful, why not say that? "Your face looks so beautiful in this light. I'd love to kiss you— would that be okay?"

You may think it sounds quaint to be talking about hugs and kisses, but that's where it starts, even if you're going to have sex on the first date—even if it's within minutes of meeting! And the principles of how to ask remain the same whether it's about kissing or genital touch or penetration.

If you set the precedent early and ask before you kiss, that sets the other person at ease that things won't happen too quickly, or without their permission. Then, if or when you get to more high-stakes acts, you're already used to talking about things and it won't seem so scary or so out of place.

If you don't start talking about sex until you're in the middle of it, sure, that could be awkward. And I think that's what most people imagine when they think about talking during sex—that it's been an entirely silent evening, simply reading each other's nonverbal cues, and then suddenly naked, in the dark, someone starts posing questions like they missed the first week of class.

Talking isn't awkward unless you make it awkward. And talking about the "small" stuff is a great way to practice, and to feel at ease when the "big" stuff comes around. So practice your communication skills as early as deciding where to meet your date, and once you're negotiating sex, it'll feel a lot easier.

NEGOTIATING MONEY

When I was sixteen years old, a college boy took me out for dinner and I let him pay. When we got back to my house and he was kissing me good night, he started getting pushy about doing other things, too, and it felt like he thought I owed him. I resolved at that point to pay my own way on dates, and for the most part I've held to that stance for the last twenty years, unless there are specific agreements around who is paying and what that means.

With one of my partners, we take turns buying dinner when we go out together. It might not end up exactly fifty-fifty, but I think it's pretty close. That way we both get to enjoy treating each other, but no one is actually taking on more of the financial burden of our dates. A friend of mine has a system where whoever makes the suggestion for a date is the one to pay.

Everyone has their own comfort levels and expectations when it comes to money. And there's no one right way of doing things. But next to sex, money is one of the most common things couples fight or miscommunicate about, so it's worth finding ways to be explicit about your wants, needs, and expectations, and to negotiate openly with your partner on these points.

Like all other expectations around sex and relationships, money should be explicitly negotiated up front. If you're expecting someone to pay for a date, make that clear. If it's important to you to pay for yourself, say that, too. If you just want to go with the flow, that's fine, but make sure you're genuinely okay with either outcome and that you're ready to deal with any assumptions that are bundled with who pays.

When it comes to dating, pay attention to how your partner manages their money. Are they living paycheck to paycheck, buying toys and treats for themselves whenever they can afford it, or are they saving for retirement or a down payment on a house? Fundamental differences like this might not matter much for someone you're dating casually, but they could cause major stress if you're planning on nesting together.

Some couples have an expectation of merging finances, while others prefer to stay independent. Some people expect to share expenses fifty-fifty while others think it's fair to be spending the same percentage of their income. Whichever seems fair or natural to you, make sure you've discussed those expectations openly with your partner before misunderstandings happen or resentments build.

A few items to consider:

Will you discuss big purchases with each other before making them? If so, what's the threshold for "big"?

How will you handle bills? A shared account? Splitting them some other way? Do you pay them as soon as the bills come in, or right before they're due?

Will one person be in charge of the finances, or will you split that chore? If so, how?

Will you check in before applying for new credit?

If you're wondering what talk of money is doing in a book about sex, it's this—money is an area where we build up expectations, and if those expectations go unvoiced, a great deal of trouble can occur. Just like my example of my date expecting something in exchange for dinner, long-term expectations can build up in partnerships around the issues of sex and money.

But just like every other issue, it's not safe to make assumptions about what taking on more of the financial load, or even giving presents, might mean. If you want finances to be part of your sexual communication and negotiation, you need to make that explicitly clear.

HANDLING JEALOUSY

In some circles, jealousy is held up as one of the best ways to show you care. In other circles, feeling or expressing jealousy is considered a personal failure. What remains consistent is that jealousy is a hot-button issue. At some point in your relationship(s), you're bound to encounter some feelings of jealousy. Personally, I don't think it's a bad thing. I think these feelings give us a chance to dig into a situation and spend time thinking about what's going on for us. Why is a particular situation troubling?

Most often, jealousy isn't a single feeling. It's an umbrella term for a whole class of feelings that could include envy or insecurity or even loneliness. Figuring out the specific details of what you're feeling will be necessary for addressing the issue.

As you're processing your feelings, there's some work you can do on your own before you talk to your partner. First, you'll want to get a clear idea of the situation. Know what's actually going on that you're reacting to. Next, make sure you take the time to acknowledge and validate your feelings. This can be as simple as taking a moment to realize that how you're feeling is normal and to make sure you don't beat yourself up about your response to the initial upset. Being mad at ourselves for feeling jealous, for example, is all too common, but that simply compounds the difficult feelings. Likewise, trying to push your feelings down or ignore them because they seem inconvenient rarely does the trick for long.

If your jealousy is about another person, see if you can spend some time with them and get to know them so that they become a real person, rather than just a scary idea. When people become more real, they often seem like less of a threat.

A trick that's been useful for me is to run the fearful thought all the way to its conclusion. If I'm worried that a partner likes something about someone else more than me, then what? Well, is that one thing all that our relationship is based on? If that one thing went away, would there still be a relationship? Generally the answer to this question is yes—relationships are complex and multifaceted and don't just hinge on one skill or shared activity.

Once you've done all the processing and self-soothing you need to do, you can decide if you'd like to talk to your partner. Sometimes we work through all the feelings on our own, and sometimes we'd like validation or reassurance from our partner, too. Make sure that you frame the conversation as being about your feelings, rather than accusing your partner of doing something wrong. And whenever possible, be clear about what you're asking for, such as compliments or reassurances.

LONG-DISTANCE RELATIONSHIPS

The saying goes that distance makes the heart grow fonder, but people who have tried long-distance relationships know that isn't always so. Yes, it can be nice to have time to miss someone. To have some anticipation between calls or visits. But missing someone can also create problems in a relationship, and it's important that you have ways to maintain your connection.

Scheduling phone calls and Skype dates are one way to stay connected. Engaging in long-distance play via text—maybe with the help of app-controlled sex toys—is another. Whatever system is right for you, just know that you can't take communication for granted. Especially when you aren't seeing someone on a regular basis.

When distance is unavoidable, spend time thinking about what it is that you need to feel connected. Like with in-person communication, quality is usually more important than quantity. Don't feel like you need to text a stream of consciousness about your day to stay connected. Instead, make sure you're talking about the important and meaningful parts of your day and your life.

Talk about your needs and your feelings, and when possible plan for the next time you'll see each other. Having a date on the calendar can make the time until then feel more bearable because you've got something to look forward to. You can use this extra time for sexy anticipation, by talking about what you'd like to do or try the next time you're together. Whether planning for a sexy event or a sexy date night at home, being reminded that you've got that intimacy coming can really help.

Being at a distance can help you hone your phone sex or sexting skills. When you're forced to use your words in this way, you may be surprised how sexy the talking can be. Talk about what you want to do the next time you're in the same room. Talk about what you'd do if you were there right at that moment. With dirty talk, it makes no sense to rush to a conclusion—it's all about the journey. So this is a great time to practice going slowly and talking about all the things you'd like to do leading up to a grand finale.

You can talk about the process of undressing each other, and the ways you'll touch. You can move slowly from tip to toe, detailing all the things you'd like to do. See how many ways you can find to build arousal and anticipation—and then when you see each other again, remember to go slowly and try all the things you talked about.

ONLINE COMMUNICATION

Online dating stresses a lot of people out. Coming up with what to say in a dating profile can feel like more pressure than writing a résumé or cover letter. And really, it's the same kind of thing—you're marketing yourself. This is also the perfect time to distill what you're all about and what you're looking for. This is the time when you can filter for all the things that are important to you, including details around sex, sexuality, and communication styles.

And when you want to catch the attention of your new Tinder match? Saying something that's clearly specific to them their profile goes a long way. So many people make generic remarks simply because they aren't trying very hard, or maybe they're copying and pasting the same one-liner to everyone. So if you're actually excited about someone, it's important to let them know why. Do you have the same hobby? The same favorite book? Do you just think they're hot?

Really engaging with what someone has put out there makes a huge difference. Most people have struggled with how to sum themselves up in just a few hundred characters, so let them know what caught your eye or that you appreciate their clever pun.

TALKING TO STRANGERS

Many of us grew up being told not to talk to strangers. Of course, now that we're adults, talking to strangers is sometimes essential. But at mixers, networking events, play parties, or even the corner bar, it can be hard to know where to start.

When people are clumped in groups, it can remind us of the high school cafeteria, and if you're anything like I was, you might rather sit alone with a book than enter that social minefield. And sometimes situations simply aren't conducive to meeting new people.

There are a few things you can do to make it easier on yourself. For one, you can learn a little about human nature. One helpful fact is that most people like talking about themselves and their interests. So it can sometimes be easier to start conversations by asking questions, especially if you have a clue as to what someone is passionate about.

At a polyamory or swingers' meet-up, you can ask about someone's experience with that lifestyle. At a kink meet-up, you can ask about someone's favorite toys, or if there are good classes or parties in the area. Even in nonsexual environments, this can work really well. Simply go to meet-ups that involve a shared passion or activity.

Rock climbing, hiking, dancing, chess, board games—whatever you're into, there's a meet-up for it. And if you go to an event that revolves around an activity, you've got a built-in conversation starter all night.

This can be a lifesaver on first dates, too. Going to a bar or restaurant that has pinball, shuffleboard, or other games gives you something to talk about. And playing the game can fill any silences that you might otherwise think are awkward.

Some meet-ups, like munches in the kink scene, come with event hosts, greeters, or facilitators. When this is the case, take advantage of it! You can message the hosts in advance and let them know that you're new, and then they can look out for you. When you get to the event, the host can then introduce you around to some of the other attendees.

Even if you haven't messaged in advance, hosts are usually happy to show new folks around. And if there isn't a party host, just walking up to whichever person seems the most confident and comfortable in the space and asking them to show you the ropes can work wonders.

TALKING TO YOUR DOCTOR

It would be great if everyone had accesses to sex-positive and fully informed health care, but unfortunately we're not there yet. That means you often have to do your own research and go to doctor visits ready to advocate for yourself. If at all possible, it's best to be completely honest with your medical providers. If you have a chance to screen your doctor before committing, you can ask about their stance on kink, open relationships, or any particulars of your situation. But ultimately, they're serving you, and you make the rules about your body and your care.

Sexual health is part of your overall well-being, so you need to be able to discuss sex with your doctor. Whether you're going to a primary-care physician or to a clinic to get tested for STIs, they'll ask questions about what activities you've engaged in. Unfortunately, doctors can be subject to the same biases as society at large, and sometimes they won't be informed about things like open relationships, kink or BDSM, or queer or transgender health issues. Sometimes they don't even have complete or accurate information about STIs.

Be prepared with your own research and information, and feel ready to insist on tests that you want to receive. If a primary-care physician is reluctant to order tests for some reason, there are labs where you can order your own tests as well as new resources for at-home testing by mail.

When it comes to kink, many people don't want to talk to their doctor about what they get up to. But sometimes it will come up anyway. If you show up to an appointment with bruises, be ready to tell your doctor, "I engage in consensual BDSM activities." Keep in mind that they're trained to ask about things like bruises, and for good reason. It's important to have that safeguard for people who are experiencing domestic violence.

Not everyone has access to the health care of their choice, but if you don't like the way you're being treated, or your doctor's stance on sexual health, I encourage you to try to move to a different clinic or doctor. Finding someone you can be open with can make a world of difference for your health and well-being.

HOW TO HANDLE REJECTION

Did you hear the story about the guy who set a goal for himself to get rejected ten times a day? He'd ask people to buy his groceries for him, to give him a ride, and he even asked people to hand over their wallets.

He was trying to get rejected often enough that he'd stop being so afraid of rejection. Sometimes this would backfire, because people were often more kind and generous than he expected and he'd get yeses when he was hoping for a no.

While I don't think you need to drag strangers into your personal growth, I do think it's important to come to terms with the possibility of rejection. Every time we ask for something, we might hear a no in response. Sometimes at a restaurant they're out of the dish you ordered, and sometimes a person you ask on a date doesn't want to go.

Our lives are full of so many yeses and noes that we probably don't even notice most of them. But when it comes to the romantic and sexual, hearing "no" seems to take on a life of its own. If a friend doesn't want to go get Thai food with us and suggests pizza instead, it doesn't usually shake our self-esteem. But if someone we have a crush on turns us down for a date, we take that very personally.

It's understandable that those things would feel different. Asking someone out makes us feel more vulnerable than asking a friend to dinner. But if we don't learn to temper our feelings around rejection (or the fear of rejection), a great deal of harm can come to ourselves and others.

Being better at accepting rejection can come from understanding the intense feelings we experience when rejected. Like any feelings we experience, it's important to acknowledge them as real and valid. And rejection is one of those feelings that's hardwired from a primal place. As social creatures, we're programmed to belong to a group. And feeling ostracized from that group is not only emotionally painful, but during earlier times in our development, it could affect our survival, too. Not only that, but along with heartbreak, rejection can activate the same areas of the brain that are affected by physical pain.

I tell you all of this not to further frighten you about the pain of rejection, but to explain that just like a stubbed toe, the pain will pass. Know that when you have these feelings, it's because that's how you're wired to feel. What you're experiencing is a natural response, and you'll come out the other side of it.

If we're so afraid of rejection that we never ask for

what we're not likely to get what we want. And if we're so upset by rejection that we lash out? Well, the news is full of stories about what happens then. But here's the great thing about rejection: we know we can trust that the person we've asked has boundaries, and it's safe to ask them for things if we know they don't feel pressured to give in.

11 Negotiation and Kink

NEGOTIATING A SCENE

Before kink play happens, it needs to be talked about. Rather than thinking of this as a chore to get through, think of it as part of the fun and a way to make sure the scene itself goes as well as possible. In fact, planning is essential to making sure everyone is safe and having fun.

Have you ever planned a vacation? Did you pick up travel guides for the places you wanted to visit, check out websites for local attractions, and start making lists of things you wanted to do? If you were traveling with other people, did you sit down and compare your lists?

Planning for play is much the same. It can involve research about the kinds of play you'd like to try, as well as actual lists of activities. And, like a vacation with other people, the input of everyone involved is needed.

Here are some steps you can take to negotiate your kink play, and some topics you need to consider.

Intentions for the scene

When we're negotiating, we usually talk about what we're going to do. But just as important is deciding how you want to feel. Do you want a scene that's about power and control? Or a scene about sensuality and pleasure? Do you want touches to be rough or tender? Do you want things to progress slowly, or do you want to be grabbed, pushed down, and fucked roughly? Even if you've covered all your bases talking about sex, bruising, bondage, and what toys are on the table, you could still end up with a big mismatch if the energy of the scene is never discussed.

Say you've decided to have a scene that includes a blindfold, light bondage, spanking, and penetrative sex. You've agreed that condoms will be used and that bruises should be avoided. Here are a couple ways that could go.

Version 1

Mira walks into the room and sees Josh sitting on the edge of the bed. She stalks over to him and shoves him so that he falls back onto the bed. As soon as he's flat, she climbs on top of him, straddling him and leaning forward to plant a rough kiss on his mouth. He makes a small noise into her mouth and she pulls away, yanking at his shirt to pull it over his head. As soon as Josh's top hits the floor, Mira has him pinned to the bed by his wrists with one of her hands, and the other is reaching to the foot of the bed to grab the coiled rope waiting there.

Mira uses her teeth to grab the bight of the rope, and then with one pull of her hand the rope uncoils across the sheets. She grabs the bight from her mouth and begins to deftly and quickly tie Josh's wrists together. As soon as they're secure, she leans farther forward, pressing her bust into Josh's face, and loops the rope around the bedpost. She kisses her way down Josh's chest, grazing her teeth across one nipple and then the other, as she continues down.

When Mira gets to Josh's belt, she gives it a yank so the buckle pops open. Two more yanks and the belt is on the floor, and his jeans soon follow. Mira doesn't show much patience for Josh's boxers, either, grabbing the waistband and pulling so that Josh's erection bounces back to slap his stomach.

Mira looks up at Josh and offers a sly grin. She appears to be sizing him up, glancing down to his feet and then bringing her eyes back up to his tied hands. Appearing to have made a decision, she reaches back down to the foot of the bed and grabs a scrap of fabric. Moving back up Josh's body, she loops the fabric behind his head, draws it across his eyes, and ties it to one side.

Josh's breathing visibly quickens when his sight is taken away. Mira runs her nails down his arms and onto his chest, then moves lower. Just when it seems like her hands will fall between his legs, she lifts them and skips to his legs. She digs her fingers in a little, squeezing the muscles of his thighs just enough to make him flinch.

Moving both hands to his left leg, she grabs the thigh and bends Josh at the knee, pulling the leg up into a ninety-degree angle and turning him half onto his side. Now his ass is exposed, and she runs her fingers quickly across his skin before pulling her hand back and bringing it down for a swat that makes Josh's flesh immediately turn pink. With only a moment's pause, her hand raises and then flies back down with another resounding smack.

The spanking continues for several moments longer, until Josh is writhing and twitching under her hand. She has mercy on him and moves his leg to lie alongside the other, soothing his warmed flesh against the soft bedspread.

Josh's cock is still hard, and now it's dripping a little bit, too. Mira smiles at the sight and grabs a condom from the nightstand. Once the package is torn open and the condom is in hand, Mira grabs Josh's erection and slides the condom down.

As soon as the condom is in place, Mira moves forward and lowers herself onto Josh. She waits only a moment to feel him settled deeply into her before she begins to move. She moves quickly, working up a rhythm that allows her to slam down onto Josh with enough force that the bed squeaks. She braces herself with hands against Josh's chest and has to be careful not to dig her nails in, despite her fingers' twitching impulse.

In just a few quick minutes, it's over, and Mira collapses onto Josh's chest as both of them start to catch their breath. When she recovers, Mira removes the blindfold, unties Josh's wrists, and pulls his body up against hers, forming a big spoon around the curve of his body.

Version 2

Josh enters the room and sees Mira sitting on the edge of the bed. He sits beside her and slides one hand into her hair, moving it out of the way and revealing the slope of her neck. He leans down to kiss her, letting his breath slide across her skin before his lips make contact. She shivers, and gooseflesh breaks out all the way down her arms.

They continue to kiss, and with a swift move, Josh

pulls Mira into his lap, never removing his lips from hers. After another long kiss, he turns her body so she's draped across his lap and supported by the bed.

Josh slides one hand into Mira's hair, weaving his fingers through her curls, and gently grabbing a handful near her scalp. With his other hand, he lifts the fabric of her nightgown, revealing her panty-clad ass. He caresses her, making the skin sensitive and bringing blood to the surface of her skin in a light blush.

When Mira starts rocking against his lap, Josh knows it's time for her spanking. He begins with gentle slaps to her ass, using an even pacing as the soft blush of her skin takes on a darker hue. Her hips press into his lap with more urgency, and he puts more force into the spanking but stays at a level of intensity he knows Mira can take for a while.

The minutes are counted in the sound of Mira's moans and the thrust of her hips. Finally, with a few hard swats, Josh finishes and positions Mira's limp, relaxed body comfortably faceup on the bed.

He pulls a length of silk fabric out of his pocket and secures her hands together, then loops the fabric around the finial on the headboard. Once she's secured, Josh takes his time exploring Mira's body with his hands and his mouth, moving her nightie as he goes and leaving more gooseflesh in his wake.

Mira makes small movements and soft sounds in response to Josh's touch, and her pupils are blown to large black discs with arousal. Josh smiles when he sees this but decides it's time to cover her lovely eyes anyway. He uses another length of the silk, and in just a moment Mira has lost the ability to watch what he's going to do next.

Josh knows that when Mira can't see what's coming, everything is felt more acutely, and he uses that to his advantage. He plays with her, pausing between one touch and the next so she can't anticipate the next sensation. This makes her squirm and writhe with anticipation between each touch.

Finally, Josh slides Mira's panties down her legs, tosses them onto the floor, and reaches for a condom from the nightstand. Once his cock is covered, he positions himself between her legs and begins the slow process of teasing her, pressing the head of his cock against her vulva but not sliding inside. Not yet. They've got all night, after all.

As you can see from these examples, knowing the facts of what's going to happen just scratches the surface of a successful negotiation. It can take some fine-tuning and some self-exploration, but understanding *how you want to feel*, rather than just *what you want to do,* makes a huge difference.

After you've decided what kind of scene you want to have, here are some additional factors to consider and to negotiate.

Likes and dislikes

In addition to intentions, it can be helpful when negotiating sex or kink to tell the other person a few things that you do and don't like. This can help build the basis for what will happen during your scene. Sometimes you may be approaching someone because of a particular skill they're known for (rope bondage, whipping, etc.), so letting the person know that's what you're interested in is helpful. Keep in mind that people want to be seen as people, not just their skill set, so be careful how you approach it, and ideally be interested in the person, too.

Will there be sex/sexual touch?

By now you know that sex can mean different things to different people. (Be sure to check chapter 3 for that point if you're skipping around.) So you know that you need to be specific about what you mean. People have very different assumptions about kink play and how it intersects with their sexuality. Some people, especially old-school kinksters, keep sex out of it. Many of the younger generation consider it integral. So when you're negotiating your scene, get crystal clear about what will and won't be involved.

- ▸ Decide if clothes are coming off or staying on.
- ▸ Decide where you can touch over clothes.
- ▸ Decide where you can touch under clothes.
- ▸ Decide if there will be penetration.
- ▸ If you are including genital touch, add in your safer-sex discussion.

Will you be using sex toys? In kink, you'll often find the top or dominant partner staying fully clothed, while the bottom or submissive might be naked or partially undressed. Sometimes toys, like a Magic Wand vibrator, might be used on bare skin or over underwear. Some people may consider this sex, and others may not. It's one of the many areas where you need to be really clear about what you mean and what you want.

Safer sex

In addition to your usual safer-sex talk that includes testing and risk information, also consider:

▸ If toys are being used, do you want them covered in a condom?

▸ With kink toys, have you discussed how they've been sanitized? Some common toy materials, like leather, can't be truly sterile.

▸ Do you want gloves used for genital or anal touch or penetration?

Substance use

If you want to play sober, say so. You can also choose a dry party to help facilitate this. If any substances are being used by anyone involved, make sure that's explicitly agreed upon.

Marks and bruises

With some forms of play, marks may be nearly inevitable. Rope suspension, for example, will almost certainly leave some bruises. Fire cupping always leaves bruises. With other toys, like whips, it's possible to use them gently, but marks are still a big risk. Other forms of play, like rope bondage on the floor, spanking, flogging, etc., may be a bit easier to control.

If you need to be absolutely sure you don't end up with marks—either because of your job, or your family, or some other reason—take this into account when deciding what kind of play to engage in, and make sure you tell your partner so they can be cautious about it as well.

Breaking skin

Beyond bruises, some kinds of play can intentionally or unintentionally break the skin. Play with needles or scalpels are some ways that people intentionally play with breaking the skin—and they're also common limits for lots of people. Whips and other toys can break the skin by accident. So it's important to note if this is something you especially want to avoid.

Power exchange

Playing with power is a big enough topic that it's got its own section later in this chapter, but don't forget to add it into your standard negotiations, too.

Safewords

It's always a good idea to have a safeword in place when you're playing with kink and BDSM. A safeword, generally, is something that you wouldn't normally say during the course of sex or play. People use safewords in part because some people like to say "no" or "stop" as part of their scene, so a different way to communicate when you're done is necessary.

Many public clubs, parties, or dungeons also have a house safeword. It's often simply "safeword" or maybe "red," but you can find this information in the party rules. When the house safeword is used, you'll have everyone's attention right away, and the party host or dungeon monitor will come and check on you. This is one of the reasons why playing in public, especially if it's with someone new, can be a safer choice.

Using the color system (green, yellow, red) is common. Green means keep going or do more, yellow means slow down, and red means stop. Some people also choose their own safeword, sometimes picking something outlandish or silly. If you do this, just make sure it's something you can remember when you need it!

In addition to safewords, using plain language is still very valuable. Unless you've specifically negotiated that you want to be able to say something like "no" without having play stop, people should be able to take you at your word.

Safewords don't replace communication! While they're a valuable tool, having safewords in place doesn't mean you can do whatever you want until you hear one. It's easy to get carried away from the top or the bottom, and sometimes people forget safewords are an option. You still need to keep an eye on your partner, and if it seems like they're struggling, pause or check in, even if a safeword hasn't been used.

Limits and boundaries

Although with many of the topics we've covered, like sex, your conversation will likely have included a discussion of limits, there may be other limits that weren't covered elsewhere. Common limits are parts of the body you never want touched (ticklish feet?) and words or names you don't want to be called.

Folks who are new to kink play often think they don't have any limits, because they're open to trying new things. But everyone has limits. Look at some fetish porn online, read some kink erotica, and watch play at your local parties. You're bound to find some things that don't appeal to you.

Injuries, health considerations, etc.

Is there anything going on with your body or your health that your partner should know about? Latex allergies, grass allergies, or even food allergies could easily come up during play, especially in public. Health issues like asthma or diabetes may also need to be noted, especially if you need to have an inhaler or other medication near at hand.

Aftercare

This has its own section later in this chapter, too, but make sure aftercare makes it onto your negotiation list. It may take playing a few times before you learn what you'll need, so let your partner know if you're not sure what you'll want after a scene.

This isn't an exhaustive list of points to negotiate, because everyone's needs and wants are unique. As you think about what points make a good and safe scene for you, consider taking notes and creating your own personal negotiation checklist.

PERSONAL NEGOTIATION CHECKLIST

To help you remember all the topics to cover in your negotiation, here is an incomplete list of things to consider.

▸ Will there be photos or videos?
▸ What words or terms will you use for each other? (Honorifics like sir, ma'am, etc.)
▸ What words or terms will you use for each other's body parts?
▸ What are each person's limits?
▸ Will there be sex?
  ▹ If so, what kind?

- ▸ What safer-sex precautions are being taken?
- ▸ What safety precautions are being taken to mitigate the risks of the kink activities?
- ▸ Will there be any substance use?
- ▸ What are each person's aftercare needs?
- ▸ Does everyone understand the risks involved?
- ▸ Does anyone have injuries or health concerns?
- ▸ Does anyone have allergies?
- ▸ What toys will be used?
- ▸ What activities will be engaged in?
- ▸ Where will the scene take place?
- ▸ When will the scene take place, and for how long?
- ▸ How do you want to feel during the scene?
- ▸ What are the top two or three things each person would like to include in the scene?
- ▸ Will there be bondage or restraint?
- ▸ Will there be marks or bruises?
- ▸ Will you be playing with pain?
  - ▹ If so, check in on a one to ten pain scale.
- ▸ Will you be using a safeword?
  - ▹ If so, what will the safeword be?

DECIDING IT WON'T WORK

Just because you've started negotiating with someone doesn't mean you have to play! Sometimes issues come up in negotiation that make it clear it isn't a good fit. That's fine. In fact, that's great. That's part of what negotiation is for. It's far better to find out at this stage that your goals and interests aren't in line and to call it quits than to go through with play, only to have it feel awkward or worse. While there are a lot of potential points that can be negotiation deal breakers, there are a few common ones, too.

If including sex or genital touch is essential to one player and off the table for the other, that's likely a bad fit and you should maybe call it quits. There are plenty of other people who want to play in the ways you do and with whom you can likely have a more successful scene.

If interest in power exchange is a mismatch, that can be another deal breaker. If one person wants to call the shots and be called by an honorific (sir, master, mistress) and the other person wants to play as equals, that can be a difficult issue to resolve.

If at any time negotiation starts to feel like an argument, walk away. You only want to play with people who are as eager to hear your limits as they are your desires. Negotiation is your chance to find out if this is going to be a good fit, and if you get a bad feeling at any time, listen to your gut.

AFTERCARE

Aftercare is an essential element of every kink scene. And what people want or need is different from person to person, so it's essential to add this point to negotiation *before* you play. One person might need time alone. Another might want snuggles and affirmations. Neither style of aftercare is right or wrong, but those two people might not be a good fit for each other, and that's better to find out in advance.

One of the great things about negotiation is that you can get creative. So maybe the person who wants to be alone can have someone stand in for them with their play partner and provide those snuggles on their behalf—if that works for their play partner.

Common aftercare needs include:
▸ Snacks
▸ Water
▸ Juice
▸ Comfy blanket
▸ Hugs/snuggles
▸ Positive affirmations
▸ Next-day check-in

And aftercare isn't just for the bottoms. All of this goes for the tops as well. Especially after rougher scenes, tops often need to hear that the bottom felt good about what happened and still likes them. Everyone should negotiate for their own needs.

Some of these items might be easy to provide in a party setting. Many events have a snack table and a water cooler. But you should still plan in advance so you don't need to walk away from your play partner to get these items when the scene ends. Try to have everything you'll need right there with you, so you can wrap the bottom up in a blanket and hand them water as soon as they're ready for it.

When it comes to length of aftercare, that's another important point to negotiate. Some people are fine after five to ten minutes, and some only want a hug. But some folks might want hours or even the whole night together. While this can be easy if you're playing at home with someone you live with, it might be harder in a party setting, or with a casual partner, so it needs to be planned in advance.

At big parties or events, some people like to pack their dance cards and move from scene to scene. This can be tricky if the people they're playing with want a lot of time together for aftercare. Again, this is a scenario where it's important to discuss needs and see if there's a way to get them met, or if this isn't a good fit. This is also a situation where outsourcing aftercare sometimes happens. Perhaps someone has a friend or partner at the event they can go to for snuggles instead of the person they just played with. Just make sure you plan this in advance, with everyone involved, so there are no hiccups finding the other person when you need them.

Even your aftercare snacks should be discussed. Some people keep chocolate in their play bag for this purpose, and that can work for many people. But some folks might have allergies or other dietary restrictions, so make sure you've figured that out.

What about check-ins the next day, or a few days later? Personally, I always like to do this. It makes me feel more at ease to know people I've played with are feeling good in their bodies and good about what happened. But not everyone wants to commit that kind of time. So make sure even these details are worked out in advance, so there aren't any hurt feelings—or unanswered text messages—in the following days.

SPECIAL CONSIDERATIONS FOR ROPE BONDAGE

There are some special considerations when negotiating rope. You need to learn to ask the right questions, such as finding out the limits of someone's flexibility and if they've had recent injuries.

People can intend to be forthcoming and still forget information that might be important to know before they're tied up. Find out if they've had any injuries at all— even injuries they don't think will matter. If someone has problems with their back, for example, a hog tie might be a terrible position for them to be in. For people with repetitive motion injuries, or injuries to their shoulders or rotator cuffs, any position that puts their arms behind their back might be problematic. Also find out if the person you plan to tie has asthma or any other breathing problems. This certainly isn't an exhaustive list—it's simply a starting point for you to talk to your partner about the ways their body does and doesn't like to move.

This is also why ongoing communication is so important. It's possible that with bondage you'll put someone in a position they've never been in before, and they might discover a problem they didn't know they had. If something is uncomfortable, the person who's tied up needs to feel empowered to speak up right away and know that changes will be made immediately—without any blame or shame.

Plan for affirmative, verbal check-ins during play. This can be as simple as "are you enjoying this?" and getting a clear, verbal yes in response. Sometimes you'll want to ask specific questions—like asking if your partner's hands are still okay or if a tie is loose enough. Be sure to ask if your partner can breathe easily.

When playing with kink in general, and bondage in particular, you need to be prepared for emotional reactions. Many people don't know how they'll react to being tied up until it happens for the first time. Some people react to the extreme vulnerability by crying. This isn't necessarily a bad thing—it could be a healthy catharsis. It's important to have had this conversation in advance so you'll know how to react and what kind of care your partner will need during and after the scene.

Depending on the tie you use, how long it lasts, and how tight it is (or if it was struggled against), rope can leave bruises or marks. Find out during negotiation if your partner is okay having lasting marks and bruises, and if so, whether they should only be visible in certain places. Rope can leave some distinctive marks, and not everyone wants to explain bruises at work or with friends and family.

Hopefully the person being tied up knows if they bruise easily, because it can be hard to predict what activity will leave a mark. Simple indentations on the wrists and ankles usually fade within an hour, but if a tie on the inner thigh digs in enough, it can leave a bruise that will last for days.

If you're playing with the same person multiple times, ask what they liked most and least about the last bondage session to help guide what you will do in the future.

HARD LIMITS

"Hard limits" is a term you hear at kink and BDSM spaces. It simply refers to a boundary or limit that you always maintain. While many limits change from day to day or partner to partner, depending what you're in the mood for, hard limits stay a bit more static and should never be pushed or tested by the person you're playing with.

We've already established that everyone has limits, but how do you figure out what they are? You can use many of the same exercises you used to figure out what you *do* want. What lines did you draw when you were considering your fantasies? Which items were on the no side of your yes/no/maybe list? All of those things are probably your hard limits, at least for now.

And your limits don't just have to be about physical

acts. You can have limits about how you want to feel, like not wanting to feel vulnerable—just make sure you also know what makes you feel that way, like bondage or blindfolds.

When you're communicating your limits, make sure the person you're talking to is paying attention and taking your limits seriously. If you get any indication that your limits won't be respected, that can be a red flag that maybe you shouldn't be playing with this person.

Here are a few things you might have hard limits around.

- Parts of your body you never want touched
- Language you aren't comfortable with
  - Body-part words
  - Names/nicknames
  - Humiliation
- Sex acts that are off-limits
- Body fluids
  - Blood
  - Ejaculate
  - Urine
  - Scat
- Breaking the skin
- Pain

NEGOTIATING POWER

The difference between topping/bottoming and dominance/submission is power. You can play with kink without playing with power, but if you're going to engage in power exchange, it should be a point of negotiation right along with the acts you're going to engage in.

Playing with power can look a lot of different ways, and

power play has its own learning curve. When you try it, you also need to negotiate the scope. Some people enjoy having power dynamics in their whole relationship (often called 24/7), and some keep it confined to their sex or kink play.

When you're starting out, or if you want to play with power for the length of a scene, it can be helpful to think about bookending. Just like the rocks or figurines that hold each end of a row of books in place, you can choose an object or ritual that helps you define the boundaries of your power play.

A common way to bookend a power exchange scene is with a collar. The person who will be submissive can kneel at the dominant's feet and have the collar put around their neck, signaling the start of the scene. At the end of the scene, the reverse can happen and the collar can be removed. This way there is a tangible reminder of when scene space is happening and when the usual relationship dynamics apply. If you don't like wearing a collar or don't want to use objects, you can also have words that you say at the beginning or end of a scene.

Keep in mind that I'm saying power *exchange* for a reason. This is because each person comes to the play on equal footing and through negotiation agrees to exchange power for the length of the scene or the relationship. When you're playing with power exchange, it's important to do your negotiating in advance, as equals. D/S or power dynamics can make it harder for people to speak up for themselves, especially for the people on the submissive side of the exchange. So make a clear time to have your negotiation and planning discussion in advance, before you take your scene roles.

If your power exchange is an element of your whole

relationship, plan regular meetings (like the state-of-the-relationship meetings mentioned earlier) where you return to your standing as equals for your check-ins and discussions.

NONVERBAL SAFEWORDS AND FEEDBACK

This is one of the only areas where I'll throw a bone to the "talking ruins the mood" camp—but not for the reasons you might think. When you're playing with kink, sometimes there's a gag involved. Other times you're playing at a loud party and regular verbal communication might not be possible. Other times, people are playing with power, or with a specific role-play scenario, and they want their communication to fit in with that fantasy.

One common tool in kink spaces is a nonverbal safeword. There are a few ways to achieve this. One common way is to have the bottom hold something in their hand, like a tennis ball or handkerchief, and have them drop it as their way of saying "yellow" or "red." If their hands are free, simply raising a hand can be a good way to get the top's attention. Stomping a foot can work as well.

For ongoing feedback during a scene, there are other ways to negotiate nonverbal communication. One can be as simple as going up on tiptoes when you need a minute to process and then returning to flat feet when you're ready for play to continue. Another version of that is being in a position where you can stick your butt out toward the other person when you want some more and move farther away when you need a minute.

YOU CAN ALWAYS SAY NO

While I hope this is abundantly clear by now, you're always allowed to say no. No matter what you've agreed to, no matter what part of play you've gotten to, you can always say no. Doesn't matter if your partner is turned on. Doesn't matter if they're a minute from orgasm. Doesn't matter if they've spent hours planning the scene or used expensive supplies. At any time, for any reason, you can say no.

Playing with kink or BDSM doesn't change these rules. Playing with power exchange doesn't change these rules. And anyone who makes you feel like there's a time when you can't say no isn't a person you should be playing with.

STICK TO THE PLAN

Although people have conflicting views on this, I think it's safest to stick to the plan for your scene and not add anything new. Of course you can always say no, or change your mind about things you agreed to. But that's about stopping or doing less than you planned. I think it's best to not increase levels of intensity or sexuality above what was agreed upon during the course of the scene.

Playing with kink gets all kinds of brain chemicals flowing, and being in those altered states can impact decision-making skills. In power-exchange play, some people refer to this as *subspace,* but that's a bit of a misnomer, because it can happen regardless of role. The same thing can happen any time you're playing with heightened states of arousal, or with pain. The effects can be similar to the use of mind-altering substances.

The good news is, if you decide there are more things you want to do, you can always make a second play date.

But you can't take back things you've done, and it's really not worth regretting your choices later.

FIRST AID

The riskier the activity you're engaging in, the more likely it is that something could go wrong. Many public parties or play spaces have people on hand to help with basic first aid, and that can add to the safety of public play. If you're playing in private, it's important to know not only the risks of the kind of play you're engaging in, but also the most likely first aid to be needed if something goes wrong. At a minimum, have a first-aid kit nearby and be ready to treat basic cuts and bruises. Ideally, get certified in CPR and basic first aid.

If something happens that requires more than basic first aid, never hesitate to call 911 (or the emergency services in your area). First responders have seen it all, and they won't be shocked by your sex or BDSM play. Get your partner the help they need right away.

RISK

Informed consent requires you to have a clear idea of the risks you're assuming with any given activity. With sex, the physical risks are often clear: STIs and pregnancy. But when it comes to kink, there can be a lot of hidden risks. Both tops and bottoms need to be fully informed. When tops know the risks of an activity they're negotiating, it's their obligation to share that information with the bottom. But sometimes tops don't know, either. Both parties are responsible for educating themselves on all the risks of the activities they want to engage in, as well as learning ways to mitigate those risks.

In the early days of the internet, BDSM forums talked about ways to differentiate kink from abuse. The core difference is consent, and they came up with the acronym SSC to stand for safe, sane, consensual. For a couple of decades, SSC was a guiding principle of kink and BDSM. You'll still commonly see it referenced in party and venue rules.

But much like the term *safe sex* evolved to *safer sex,* SSC has been updated. Many kinksters pointed out that the activities they were engaging in were never really safe. In an effort to more accurately describe the kink ethos, the term *RACK,* for risk-aware consensual kink, was born. Replacing *safe* with *risk aware* is meant to acknowledge that none of these activities are truly safe, but when engaging in them within a consensual BDSM context, all participants are aware of the risks.

These days the acronyms live alongside each other, with many parties and venues choosing to adopt one or the other. The connotations imply that the RACK parties are sometimes edgier or riskier and are more likely to include activities that are considered to have higher risk, like play that breaks the skin (needles, hooks) or includes fire. Many players (myself included) consider rope suspension a high-risk activity as well. From spanking to cutting, every activity has *some* risk, and it's up to you to learn about it and decide if it's something you're comfortable with.

From books to classes to conferences, there are many ways to learn more about the kinds of kink you're interested in. So be sure to do your research the same way you would when new to any activity. As a potential bonus, classes and conferences are a great way to meet fellow kinksters. And the likelihood that someone is interested in safety is a bit higher when you meet them at a class. At a minimum, it's easier to start the conversation when you've both just heard the same information.

SCENES GONE WRONG

Even with the best of intentions, and clear communication and negotiation in place, things can and do go wrong in kink and BDSM. That's part of the risk you're accepting when you play this way, and hopefully you also know in advance about the specific risks of what you're doing. But accidents happen, and it's important to have some idea of how you want to handle them before you're in the moment.

When BDSM scenes go wrong, it can be anything from an intentionally crossed boundary (which may be assault or abuse) to an honest accident. We aren't talking legal definitions here, but your response to the incident might be different depending on the intention.

If someone ignores your safeword or continues playing after you've said stop, there's a problem. Ignoring your no is never okay. These blatant consent violations may have legal consequences, and they're not the kind of problems we're addressing here. What this section is meant to address is scenes gone wrong that were accidents or miscommunications. There's no excuse for intentional boundary crossing or abuse.

Regardless of your role—top, bottom, dominant, or submissive—things can happen that you don't feel good about. All too often we only consider the bottom or submissive when it comes to boundary crossings, but tops and dominants have boundaries, too, and they're no less important.

If things have gone wrong at a party, you may want to tell the party host or venue owner, even if it was accidental. (If someone acted in a way that was malicious, or with complete disregard to consent or to your safety, you may want to tell local hosts and organizers, no matter where the incident occurred.) Different communities have different ways of handling these issues. Of course, many times people don't feel safe or comfortable speaking out about the things that have happened to them. Only you can decide what's right for you.

One reason you might want to share about your scene gone wrong is so that other people can learn from your experience. In a general way, you're helping other people understand that these activities are risky. And if there was a specific problem (equipment failure, etc.), you might be able to keep other people from having the same issue.

Immediately after a scene gone wrong isn't necessarily the best time to talk about it. It's important for the parties involved to assess what they need, both in the moment and for follow-up. If there's anger or hurt feelings, the people involved might want support from someone else in the immediate aftermath rather than the person they were playing with.

If you don't talk about things right away, make sure to set a concrete time to do so. If there's an apology to be made, it should be done as quickly and sincerely as possible. It can also be helpful to talk about what happened and figure out where things went wrong. Was there an unclear boundary or limit? Was there a misunderstanding of technique? Knowing why things went wrong can help make sure it doesn't happen again, either with this pairing or with future partners.

Aftercare often involves reassurances that you like and trust your partner, especially when there was heavy play. When something goes wrong, aftercare—and these assurances—can be especially important. But sometimes it takes a while to get there. While feelings are hurt, and before things are repaired, you might need to get support from other people.

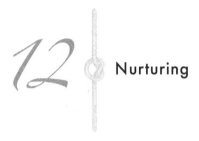

Nurturing

SELF-CARE

WHILE YOU'RE WORKING ON MAINTAINING OR improving connection with a partner or partners, make sure you're also taking care of yourself. Relationship issues can feel all consuming, and before you know it, you can fall into patterns that aren't ideal for you. Or you can fall out of good habits. Make sure you're always prioritizing yourself and your own well-being.

This is something I tell clients when they start working with me. Digging into issues around sex, sexuality, and relationships can bring up lots of feelings you'll need to address. If nothing else, you're likely to feel more emotional or more vulnerable during the process. This can make it especially important that you have a plan for taking care of yourself.

Many of us struggle with eating well, sleeping enough, and getting enough exercise even during the best of times, let alone when we're feeling strained or stressed. So it can be valuable to plan for this kind of care alongside any planning you do around trying new kinds of relationships, sex, or kink.

Know what makes you feel your best, and also know what works as self-soothing when you're feeling worn thin. Have a list of things that you can try so you don't have to think about it when you're at your lowest point. Anything from time in a hot tub or bath to getting a massage, taking a nap, or going for a walk might make this list. There are no wrong answers—you just need to know what works for you, and you need to plan for the time it takes to do these things on top of your normal schedule.

CAMPSITE RULE

Originally a motto for scouting troops, the "campsite rule" refers to leaving camping grounds in as good a shape as you found them, if not better. So, no leaving trash around or destroying the habitat. Dan Savage adapted this rule for relationships, in his case usually using it when one partner is significantly older than the other. The way he says it, when one partner has more experience, it's their ethical obligation to take extra care of their younger or less experienced partner. I don't disagree.

But I'd take it a step further—why not aim for this in all relationships? Most of us have some kind of baggage from past relationships, or from simply existing in a sex-negative, body-shaming culture. We can work on healing those wounds, one person at a time, by lavishing our partners with positive reinforcement.

Tell them you love their bodies. Be receptive to their sexual interests and kinks. Show that it's possible to have a relationship with open and honest communication.

Don't become the ex someone tells horror stories about— have the kind of relationship where you can stay friends, even after a breakup. Be the kind of partner who sets an example for how relationships can be.

This doesn't mean there's never conflict. It doesn't mean the relationship lasts forever. But we can be kind and nurturing to each other, even when there are fundamental mismatches that mean romantic connections aren't possible. I'm friends with most of my past partners, and it's incredibly fulfilling to maintain connections with people who have been important to me, even when the sexual or romantic aspects of our dynamic have come to an end.

There's something to be learned from every relationship and connection, even if what you're learning is what *doesn't* work for you. A relationship that ends doesn't have to be a failure. Too much of our culture treats ended relationships as an embarrassment we have to put behind us. But that's just another facet of our unhelpfully goal-oriented society, where there's a narrow view of success.

So wherever you can, help pick up the litter left behind by previous partners, and leave everyone with a tidy campsite if and when you leave.

DATE FOLLOW-UPS AND CHECK-INS

Aftercare isn't just for kink! It's lovely to follow up with someone after a date and let them know you had a good time (as long as that's true!). This can also be a way to extend the good feelings of the date and to start planning for the next one.

This is one area where common dating advice really goes off the rails and encourages harmful game playing.

Advice givers act like there's a one-size-fits-all answer for how soon to get in touch after a date or how long to wait before you answer a text message (or email, or phone call).

But any advice that says there's one way to do things is encouraging you to be less than genuine. And ultimately, that doesn't serve anyone. If you're following rules prescribed in a book or an article online, you'll ultimately not be getting your needs met.

If you feel inspired later that night, or the next day to tell someone you had a lovely time, do it. If the other person doesn't like that kind of contact, that's a conversation to be had. But ultimately if you're a higher-contact person, you want to find someone with the same style rather than tamp down your own needs to fit their preferences. That isn't sustainable in the long run.

If there are certain kinds of contact you'd like to receive, be sure to ask for them. Asking for someone to check in when they get home safely is a nice gesture and provides a built-in follow-up. You can also talk about parts of the date you especially enjoyed and things you'd like to do next time.

PLAY WITH ANTICIPATION

Having special events and planned dates to look forward to is a great way to maintain connection and build anticipation when life is busy. But you can go beyond simply scheduling a date night and actively build anticipation all day, or even all week.

Find creative ways to leave each other notes, send texts throughout the day, or plan the outfits and toys you'll use. Finding ways to plan that build excitement and anticipation helps quell the fears that scheduling makes things boring. Not only that, it'll make the event itself hotter and ensure you'll look forward to the next scheduled date.

If you live together, you can also step up the compliments and flirting around the house. Tell your partner how cute they look first thing in the morning, or fresh out of the shower. Give them an extra squeeze or kiss when they're out the door to work in the morning, and say how eager you are to see them that night. We all want to feel wanted. Sometimes all it takes is saying the things you already think (and maybe take for granted) out loud.

KEEP EACH PERSON SPECIAL

Having special things you do with a partner, or say to a partner, is just one way to differentiate that relationship from the other connections in your life. This can be anything from calling them pet names to saying good night in a particular way to bringing them their favorite flower now and then.

If you have multiple partners, it might be helpful to have unique rituals associated with each partner to help each connection feel special. This can be everything from using a different set of sheets to burning different scents of incense to playing different music.

Just like asking someone how their body likes to be touched, it can help to ask someone what makes them feel special. What kind of check-ins do they enjoy? How do they like to hear that you're thinking of them?

What can you do to maintain connection throughout this whole process of exploration? Don't forget to keep doing all the things that are already working, and don't let sexual exploration become such a full-time job that you don't go see a movie now and then.

It's important not to let other aspects of life and relationships suffer when the focus is shifted to sex, because as wonderful as sex is, it's only one aspect of our relationship with ourselves and with other people.

ALWAYS A WORK IN PROGRESS

Every section of this book is about ways to explore and fine-tune your sexual experience. There isn't any set goal you're trying to reach, and there is no perfect sex life to achieve. Like all areas of our life, sex can (and should) remain a work in progress our entire lifetimes.

We will continue learning things about ourselves, about the kinds of sex that are possible, and about our partners. That's part of what's amazing about sexuality and part of the fun! There's always something new to look forward to and something new to try.

And having that outlook of learning and growing will serve you well because our own bodies change over time, too, so we need to be ready to keep figuring out what works for us as our own bodies and interests evolve.

Keep an open mind.

Try new things.

Have fun.

ODDS AND ENDS • RESOURCES

Websites:

Autostraddle's Yes/No/Maybe List: https://www. autostraddle.com/you-need-help-here-is-a-worksheet-to-help-you-talk-to-partners-about-sex-237385/

Betty Martin: https://bettymartin.org

Brené Brown: http://brenebrown.com

Caffyn Jesse: http://www.erospirit.ca

CDC information on oral sex risk: https://www.cdc.gov/ std/healthcomm/stdfact-stdriskandoralsex.htm

Cuddle Party: http://www.cuddleparty.com

CripConfessions: http://cripconfessions.com

Cunning Minx, poly weekly podcast: http://polyweekly .com

HeyEpiphora, sex toy reviews: https://heyepiphora.com

Jiz Lee's article on safer sex in queer porn, with an STI chart (NSFW): http://jizlee.com/safer-sex-in-queer-porn-and-the-condom-debate/

Kate Kenfield http://www.katemccombs.com

Marcia Baczynski: https://www.askingforwhatyouwant .com

Mollena Lee Williams-Haas: http://www.mollena.com

Planned Parenthood STI information: https://www .plannedparenthood.org/learn/stds-hiv-safer-sex

Poly Role Models: http://polyrolemodels.tumblr.com

Safety information for rope bondage: Remedialropes.com

SexAbled: https://www.sexabledwithrobinwb.com

Scarleteen's info on STIs: http://www.scarleteen.com/article/sexual_health/sti_risk_assessment_the_cliffs_notes

Tristan Taormino: http://tristantaormino.com

Online shopping:

JoEllen Notte's superhero sex toy store list, or, how to find an awesome sex toy store near you: http://www.redheadbedhead.com/superhero-sex-shops/

Good Vibrations, sex toys and lube: https://www.goodvibes.com/s

SheVibe, sex toys and lube: https://shevibe.com

SheBop, sex toys and lube: http://sheboptheshop.com

Twisted Monk, rope bondage: https://www.twistedmonk.com

Lucky Bloke, condoms: https://luckybloke.com

Sex-positive therapist resources:

Therapists can be an incredible resource when you need some extra support. It's also important to find a therapist who meets your needs. You get to be choosy! Call around and interview potential therapists and make sure you like where they stand. You can ask about everything from their modalities to their familiarity with different sexualities and relationship structures. If you know you want someone sex positive and/or kink aware, here are a few places where you can start looking.

AASECT: https://www.aasect.org/referral-directory

Open List: http://openingup.net/open-list/

Kink Aware Professionals: https://www.ncsfreedom.org/key-programs/kink-aware-professionals-59776

Books:

As Kinky as You Wanna Be: Your Guide to Safe, Sane and Smart BDSM by Shanna Germain

Come as You Are: The Surprising New Science that Will Transform Your Sex Life by Emily Nagoski PhD

Curvy Girl Sex: 101 Body Positive Positions to Empower Your Sex Life by Elle Chase

The Ethical Slut: A Practical Guide to Polyamory, Open Relationships, and Other Freedoms in Sex and Love by Janet W. Hardy and Dossie Easton

Femalia, edited by Joani Blank

Girl Sex 101 by Allison Moon and kd diamond

More Than Two: A Practical Guide to Ethical Polyamory by Franklin Veaux and Eve Rickert

Nonviolent Communication: A Language of Life by Marshall Rosenberg, PhD

Perv: The Sexual Deviant in All of Us by Jessie Bering

Sex Outside the Lines: Authentic Sexuality in a Sexually Dysfunctional Culture by Chris Donaghue PhD

She Comes First: The Thinking Man's Guide to Pleasuring a Woman by Ian Kerner

SM 101: A Realistic Introduction by Jay Wiseman

The Threesome Handbook: A Practical Guide to Sleeping With Three by Vicki Vantoch

The Ultimate Guide to Sexual Fantasy: How to Have Incredible Sex with Role Play, Sex Games, Erotic Massage, BDSM Play and Much, Much More by Violet Blue

Porn:

Watching porn can be a great way to explore sexual interests, either alone or with a partner. If you're not sure where to start, here are a few suggestions.

Crash Pad/Pink Label
Erika Lust
Aorta Films
amateurporn.com
Beautiful Agony
CherryStems
Four Chambers
TrenchCoatX
Spit.exposed

Erotica:

When you're using erotica to try out new fantasies, anthologies are a great resource. There are even anthologies of short shorts so that you're not committing to more than a couple of pages of reading to decide if you're intrigued by a certain kind of sex or kink. Here are a few suggestions of where to start:

The Big Book of Orgasms: 69 Sexy Stories
The Big Book of Bondage
Sudden Sex: 69 Sultry Short Stories
Bondage Bites: 69 Super-Short Stories of Love, Lust and BDSM

Beyond these suggestions, I wholeheartedly recommend anything written or edited by Rachel Kramer Bussel, Shanna Germain, Kristina Wright, and Alison Tyler.

Safer-sex details

Information about sexual health should be easy to come by, but that's not always the case. Schools don't usually do a good job, and all too often our regular doctors don't, either. Planned Parenthood is a wonderful resource for information about STIs and other sexual-health issues. They're also a source for testing and related counseling. See their website for updated and timely information.

When it comes to figuring out what infections you can get from which activities, it comes down to part statistics and part guesswork. That's because when they conduct surveys of people who are getting STI tests, the participants have usually engaged in a number of different activities, and so the exact transmission can rarely be pinpointed.

Still, we have plenty of information to know that any time you're engaging in skin-to-skin contact with another person, there is a potential risk of STI transmission, and that risk greatly increases when there's a sharing of fluids.

For more information on the following sexually transmitted infections and what activities can transmit them, visit Planned Parenthood (www.plannedparenthood.org) and the Centers for Disease Control and Prevention (www.cdc.gov).

- ▶ Chlamydia
- ▶ Gonorrhea
- ▶ Syphilis
- ▶ Herpes (HSV 1 and HSV 2)
- ▶ HIV and AIDS
- ▶ HPV (human papillomavirus)
- ▶ Trichomoniasis (trich)
- ▶ Hepatitis B

- ▸ Genital warts
- ▸ Molluscum contagiosum
- ▸ Pubic lice (crabs)
- ▸ Scabies

When you go to your doctor or to a clinic to be tested, be clear about which tests you'd like to receive. Unfortunately, it sometimes comes down to what's covered by insurance. If money is a factor, Planned Parenthood offers tests on a sliding scale, and many county health departments offer low-cost testing as well.

In some places testing for HSV 1 and 2 has fallen out of favor because of the chance of false positives, and because many doctors don't consider it a serious health concern. If you'd like to get this test and your doctor doesn't want to do it, you can sometimes order it at a lab by paying out of pocket.

The other important thing to know is that some infections, like chlamydia and gonorrhea, can be location specific—meaning that you can have them orally (in your throat) or anally, and they won't appear in urine tests. You need to ask for location-specific swabs, and this is something else most doctors won't offer and often don't even know about.

For these reasons and more, being fully informed and being ready to advocate for yourself is essential when it comes to sexual health and well-being.

Although the above mostly details the ways these infections can be transmitted sexually, there can also be risk during kink play that breaks the skin, or where blood is drawn. Any time you're exposed to someone else's blood, you're at high risk for a variety of infections.

SUPPLIES

Lube: Lube makes everything better! I'm shocked when students or clients tell me they've never used lube or when I go home with somebody and they don't have lube. (Luckily I usually have a few packets in my purse.) My personal favorites are Sliquid water-based lube and Uber-lube for if/when you want silicone lube.

Like all things relating to sex, there is tons of bad and misleading information about lube out there. For one thing, it doesn't mean a failure of anyone's body or technique to use lube. Not all bodies self-lubricate, and certain body parts never self-lubricate! If you're trying anal sex or giving a hand job to a penis, there's never self-produced lubricant. And even vaginas that self-lubricate can often use some extra help.

Unfortunately there are a lot of bad lubes on the market. Your doctor may suggest something that isn't great, and most of the lubes you'll find at the drugstore aren't great for you, either. There are a lot of ingredients you want to avoid, including glycerin, glucose, and their derivatives, which can cause yeast infections. More ingredients to avoid include parabens, petroleum or petroleum-derived ingredients, propylene glycol, and chlorhexidine. Just like when you're at the grocery store, you're going to have to read the ingredients.

A few more lube caveats: oil degrades latex, so you can't used oil-based lube, including things like coconut oil, if you're going to use condoms or barriers in your sex. Also, silicone lube degrades silicone sex toys, so if you're using silicone toys or dildos, be sure to use water-based lube.

Condoms: Condoms come in a variety of sizes and materials to suit many different bodies and purposes. They're an essential safer-sex supply when you're engaging with a bio penis, and they're also very helpful for using over shared sex toys.

Gloves: You may associate gloves with the doctor's office more than the bedroom, but gloves are a fantastic safer-sex supply. They're available in both latex and nitrile, so you can find a material that works for you. Gloves provide safety when engaging in hand sex and they also make cleanup a lot easier. Not only that, but they help smooth rough edges like calluses and fingernails, which could otherwise cause microtears on delicate tissues, opening people up to possible infections.

You can get gloves in a variety of colors, which is not only fun but a trick that can be used to color code hands for different uses (one for a vulva, one for the anal area—to avoid cross contamination) or to color code between multiple partners during multiperson sex.

Dental dams: Dental dams are sheets of latex or polyurethane you can use to cover a vulva or anus for performing oral sex. You can also make one by cutting open a condom or a glove.

Bondage rope: If you want to start playing with rope bondage, get rope that's made for that purpose. Most of what you'll find at hardware stores isn't good for your skin or isn't safe to use.

Kink toys: You can find lots of things around the house or kitchen to use as "pervertables" things you're using outside their usual context. Wooden spoons and hair-brushes make fantastic, if very mean, paddles. You can also find toys around the house for sensation play. If you decide you want more than that, like restraints, floggers, candles, or more, be sure to go with reputable makers and retailers to assure you're getting high-quality and body-safe products.

Sex toys: Sex toys are a fabulous addition to anyone's solo or partnered sex. Regardless of your gender or genitals, there's something for you. Shopping from any of the sex-positive retailers in the resources section is a great way to start, but here are a few things to think about and look out for.

Not all sex toys are created equal! Less-reputable retailers and online stores often carry toys that are not body safe. Jelly materials can leach chemicals that aren't good for you and should be avoided. Look for toys made from one hundred percent silicone or other body-safe materials. You can read up about sex toys in the links provided in the resources section.

GLOSSARY

Aftercare: Providing care to someone after a kink scene.

Analingus or Rimming: Refers to using the mouth and tongue on the anus.

Barrier: Any form of physical protection, like condoms or dental dams.

BDSM: For this acronym, some letters do double duty. Bondage and discipline, domination and submission, sadism and masochism.

Cis: the commonly used shortened form of Cisgender, which is the designation for people whose gender identity corresponds with the one assigned at birth.

Dominant/submissive: Similar to top and bottom, but this time with a power-exchange element. The submissive gives power to the dominant for the negotiated space of the scene. Some people also have an overarching D/S dynamic for their entire relationship.

Electrical play: Using kink toys made for electricity, like violet wands or TENS units.

Exhibitionism: Getting sexual pleasure from being seen or watched.

Fetish: The true definition refers to something that must be present in order to achieve sexual gratification, but the word is often used colloquially as interchangeable with kink.

Fire cupping: cupping is a form of traditional medicine, of which fire cupping is one variety, that has been practiced around the world for thousands of years. In the case of fire cupping, fire is used to create a vacuum inside the cup being used before placing the cup on the skin, typically on the back. That vacuum then pulls the skin up into the cup. This practice leaves distinctive round bruises and due to the intense sensations experienced it is also practiced in the kink community.

Fisting: Fisting is when you put your whole hand, up to the wrist, into the orifice of your choice. In my case, it was vaginal fisting.

Frottage: Sexual rubbing, nonpenetrative sex, with or without clothes on.

Kink: Often used to refer to sexual practices considered unconventional, in my experience, "kink" refers to anything just a little taboo to the person saying something is kinky. Sometimes used colloquially to refer to anything someone is into sexually. People who are asexual may also practice kink. The motivations and rewards for these behaviors are different for everyone.

Masochist/masochism: Deriving sexual pleasure from receiving pain. From the writer Leopold von Sacher-Masoch.

Pegging: Coined by a Dan Savage reader, pegging usually refers to a woman using a strap-on dildo to anally penetrate a man.

Play: Whatever form of sex or kink you're engaging in with someone.

Play partner: The person you're engaging in kink or sex activities with.

Relationship escalator: Most often seen in writing about polyamory or relationship anatomy, the relationship escalator refers to the societally prescribed way a relationship is expected to progress, from dating, to living together, to marriage, to children, etc.

Sadist/sadism: Deriving sexual pleasure from giving pain. From the writer Marquis de Sade.

Sex positive: A term popularized by Carol Queen[8] that encompasses a wide range of beliefs about how both individuals and society can relate to sex and sexuality in a healthy way. Being sex positive means being nonjudgmental and nonshaming. Sex positivity encompasses any sexual expression, including asexuality.

---

8   Carol Queen, "What Sex-Positivity Is—And Is Not," *Good Vibes* (blog), March 4, 2014, https://goodvibesblog.com/sex-positivity/.

Scene: Usually in relation to kink, a scene refers to the time when kink play is taking place. Can also be used more generally to refer to the whole kink community, as in, "the kink scene."

Strap-on: Using a harness that holds a dildo to your pelvis. Can be worn or used by people of any gender. There are varieties that allow space for a bio penis. There are also strap-on harnesses that can be worn on other parts of the body, like the thigh or chest.

Switch: Someone who switches between top and bottom, or dominant and submissive roles, whether with the same or different partners.

Top/bottom: Used in both the queer and kink communities, top refers to the person giving sensation or the person "doing," and bottom refers to the person receiving sensation. However, bottoming is not necessarily a passive role.

Unicorn: A slang term used to refer to a potential third party for a threesome. Usually in reference to a bisexual woman, but can be applied to any gender. The reference pokes fun at the idea that a young, attractive, bisexual woman who will be equally attracted to both parties in a couple will appear for a threesome, and then go away, without having any needs of their own. Impossible, hence "unicorn." Couples who are looking for a third in a way that treats people like objects are often called unicorn hunters.

Voyeurism: Getting sexual pleasure from watching others.

ABOUT THE AUTHOR

STELLA HARRIS is changing the way people experience their sex lives. As a certified intimacy educator and sex coach, she gives people the tools and confidence to explore their sexuality safely and free of shame. A national and international speaker, Harris teaches everything from pleasure anatomy to communication skills, kink, and BDSM.

Harris has been widely quoted in the media, and she's made guest appearances on numerous podcasts, including *Playboy Radio*. Her articles have appeared across the Web including in *Cosmopolitan* and *Kinkly,* where she's been honored as a sex-blogging superhero for four years running. She authors the *Willamette Week*'s sex column, "Humptown," and her fiction appears in the books *As Kinky as You Wanna Be, The Big Book of Bondage,* and more than a dozen other collections.

Find Harris around the web on her website, www.stellaharris.net, on Twitter, @stellaerotica, and on Instagram, @stellaharriserotica.

Printed in the United States
By Bookmasters